Extreme Fat Smash Diet

extreme
FAT smash
DIET

Ian K. Smith, M.D.

St. Martin's Griffin ≈ New York

www.stmartins.com

Library of Congress Cataloging-in-Publication Data
  Smith, Ian, 1969–
  The extreme fat smash diet / by Ian K. Smith—1st ed.
    p. cm.
  ISBN-13: 978-0-312-37120-3
  ISBN-10: 0-312-37120-9
  1. Reducing diets.   I. Title.

RM222.2. S6221 2007
613.2'5—dc22

                                        2006102537

Design by Fritz Metsch

10 9 8 7 6

Dedication

I want to dedicate this book to Pamela El, Rachel Jacobs, and Angela Barnhart. Three strong, beautiful, and committed women who, like hundreds of other SMASHERS, went on the program and not only lost a significant amount of weight, but changed their lives forever. I will always be inspired by their determination and zest for a long, healthy, and happy life.

Contents

Acknowledgments

There were many people who helped me organize my thoughts and even served as "test cases" for this book. I'd like to thank Rena Cherry, Dana Smith, Sita Silva, Elizabeth Beier, Michelle Richter, Steve Cohen, Matthew Shear, Jonathan and Shelly Cardi, Pam El, Michelle House, Dr. Sharon Lieteau, and, of course, the queen of my life, Triste Lieteau Smith.

Extreme Fat Smash Diet

CHAPTER 1

Extreme Fat Smash Philosophy

EXTREME: going to great lengths or beyond normal limits

That's the *Merriam-Webster's Dictionary* definition of "extreme" and the one I like most when thinking about the core principles of this exciting weight-loss program. Some may see the word "extreme" and cringe because they associate it with pain, while others will want to investigate further because they're curious or experience a rush of adrenaline as their mind immediately prepares itself for an exciting challenge. It's my hope that when people see the words **EXTREME FAT SMASH,** they will be both curious and ready for a challenge.

Most of us travel through life in what I call the safety zone, whether it's always making conservative and predictable career moves or making personal decisions without risk and the possibility of loss. There's nothing wrong with this philosophy for most people. But for someone who wants to achieve *greatness* and accomplish extraordinary things, living in the safety zone is not going to deliver the desired results. **EXTREME FAT SMASH** is for people who are determined to reach what they might've considered unthinkable success in a weight-loss journey. The idea is simple: if you want big results, then you'll have to push yourself beyond the normal limits to attain them.

EXTREME FAT SMASH is not a fad diet. The science behind the program is not only credible but also well tested. Many of us diet experts have preached for a long time that it's best to lose weight slowly, because gradual, consistent weight loss increases the likelihood that you will lose more weight and have a greater chance of keeping that weight off. I still hold fast to that viewpoint. So if you're trying to lose 50 to 100 pounds or even more, it's more practical for you to embark on a weight-loss program that will deliver this type of gradual weight loss. You would benefit tremendously from my original FAT SMASH DIET. That 90-day program will guide you to significant weight loss spread over an appropriate amount of time. But if you're trying to lose 10 to 25 pounds in a short period of time, you want to do it in a healthy manner, and you want to keep those pounds off for good, then EXTREME FAT SMASH is the program for you.

Many diets promise tremendous weight results in a short period of time, and some of them actually deliver. But the manner in which these results were achieved was often unsafe, medically risky, and short lasting. What I have set about to do is something that millions of dieters have been asking for, yet the experts said it either couldn't be done or shouldn't be attempted. EXTREME FAT SMASH is a plan that will help you reach those quick results, but you'll get them by eating healthy foods and following a specific exercise program that will help condition your heart, muscles, and lungs. You will not be required to take any dangerous weight-loss supplements or eat foods that could eventually prove harmful to your health. Not only will you lose weight on this program, but you will learn the values of nutritionally powerful foods and how to create portion-controlled meals.

I would be dishonest if I did not tell you that there will be moments on this diet that you will be discouraged or tired or even ready to throw in the towel. This is completely normal and expected. Why? Because you'll be pushing your mind and body beyond the normal limits. Here's an exercise to help you find inner resources: stand in front of a mirror and look as deeply as you can into your eyes for 90 seconds. Don't blink, don't move your eyes, blur out everything else in the mirror, and block out all of the noises you hear. Focus only on your eyes. This exercise will teach you how to reach into your soul and find that inner strength that will allow you to continue your march forward even when things seem to be getting tough. What you're looking at in the mirror is your essence, your drive, your determination to make a big change in your life.

SOMETIMES WE MUST GO THROUGH DARKNESS TO REACH THE LIGHT.

EXTREME FAT SMASH is a very specific diet, and it must be, because you're asking your body to undergo some rapid changes in a very short period of time. Because the time line is so tight, it's critical that you follow the program *as written*. It has been thought through and tested to give you your best chance of obtaining optimal results. If you're determined to reach your goal and you're tired of learning the hard way that all of those advertised shortcuts never deliver on their promises, then **EXTREME FAT SMASH** is the program for you.

As you work your way through the three cycles of the program, it's important to remember that you are eating to satisfy hunger, not eating because the food is there or to the point of being stuffed. Your schedule will be set up so more food is always coming soon, so train yourself not to overdo it at any meal or snack!

CHAPTER 2

Why It Works

There's nothing magical about a good diet and no tricks or easy ways out, either. **EXTREME FAT SMASH** is based on sound scientific principles and thoughtful research, as well as many years of shared dieting experiences. But a diet is only as good as the dieter's execution of the plan. Dieting is like war. If a battalion of soldiers goes into battle with a great plan, but once they get to the battlefield decide to deviate from the plan without good reason, then that plan is no longer effective. No plan works if it isn't followed. The biggest two reasons outside of the diet design itself why **EXTREME FAT SMASH** will work are (1) you know it will work and (2) you follow the plan vigorously.

Believing in something—whether it's a dieting plan, your ability to pass an exam, or get a promotion at work—is extremely important not just for success on **EXTREME FAT SMASH,** but for life in general. You've heard of the phrase "mind over matter." Well, there's a lot more to those three words than you think. Belief is as much about your internal conviction as it is about your mental determination to get the job done. Is this program going to push you? Yes. Is this program going to ask you to work hard? Yes. But if you believe in the program and your abilities, then you will achieve tremendous success.

EXECUTION

One of the things that makes me proudest of **EXTREME FAT SMASH** is the feedback from those who have done it. My vision for the program is what most resonated with the **SMASHERS.** They were happy that they could actually eat real food, not feel hungry between meals, maintain high levels of energy throughout the day, and avoid feeling like they were on a "diet." In order for any program to work it must be designed so that people can actually follow the program and incorporate it into their everyday life. Designing a good plan is only half the battle; the other half is someone being able to execute the plan.

EXTREME FAT SMASH is designed so that you will not have to do anything drastic in your daily schedule to accommodate the plan's eating schedule and exercise program. Yes, you will have to make some changes. You will have to spend a little more time thinking ahead and organizing your day, and you might have to replace some of that TV leisure time with a 40-minute workout, but the plan is designed for all types of lifestyles, from the home-based soccer mom to the corporate executive who spends enormous amounts of time in meetings or traveling. I've made the daily eating and exercise requirements aggressive but realistic, so that you can go on living your life with as little disturbance as possible and still meet your goals by the time you reach the end of the program. Just remember, organization is key. So the last thing you should do every night before climbing into bed is to look at the next day's plan and think about what you're going to have to do to make it work.

PORTION CONTROL

If you have ever been on a diet before or heard any expert talk about diets, you've heard the term "portion control." The reason why you've heard it so much is that it's important, it makes sense, and it works. Part of the reason why **EXTREME FAT SMASH** helps you obtain the results you want is that it teaches you about portion control. But you don't learn by reading through dense medical journal articles or sitting in front of a blackboard listening to a boring lecture. You learn by doing. You learn by following the program. There's nothing groundbreaking about the fact that Americans consume too many calories at each meal. Our society has become one of jumbo-sized portions and it has had a direct effect on our waistlines and our overall health.

Even if your diet isn't extremely healthy, just limiting the size of the portions you consume can have a dramatic effect on your weight. I've consulted many people who had unhealthy diets but decided to make one change in their eating life: reducing the size of their meals. Not only did they find that eating smaller meals still satisfied

Dr. Ian's Tip

If you want to stop yourself from eating a large serving of food, then cut it in half. On the half that you're not going to eat, sprinkle something you don't like, such as pepper, ketchup, mustard—anything that will ruin the flavor and stop you from eating it.

their hunger, they lost 10–15 pounds in a year without making any other change.

SMART CHOICES

One of the major reasons so many people fail on diets is that they never learn the art of making smart choices. It's not that they don't *want* to do the right thing. They just don't know *how* to do it and the diet they've picked never teaches them how. Every day you make hundreds of small decisions that have an impact on whether you're going to gain weight or lose weight. One reason **EXTREME FAT SMASH** works is that you'll quickly learn how to make the right choices, so much so that it becomes second nature.

What often separates those who are successful on a weight-loss program from those who are not are small decisions made throughout the day. For example, deciding to use low-fat milk in your cereal instead of whole milk. How about choosing mixed berries for dessert instead of ice cream that has five times the number of calories? Each individual decision doesn't have much of an impact, but when you add those decisions up at the end of the day—or at the end of the week—there's a big difference between the dieter who made good decisions 80 percent of the time and the dieter who made good decisions only 35 percent of the time. The goal of this program is to get you into that 80 percent group. In order to do that, keep in mind that small bad decisions have a cumulative effect. At the end of the week they can be the determining factor in whether you lose 2 pounds or 4.

FIBER

Most people have heard about fiber, but they don't know what it is, where it comes from, and why it's important for our health. If you know these answers, you'll be well on your way to making smart choices that will not only help you **SMASH** the fat but also improve your overall health.

EXTREME FAT SMASH advocates increasing your fiber intake because of all of its potential health benefits. Fiber is a complex carbohydrate (big-sized sugar) that your body is unable to digest or absorb into the bloodstream. Fiber is what gives plants their shape. Celery has a rigid stalk because of fiber. In fact, fiber is found only in foods that come from plants, such as fruits, vegetables, legumes (beans, peas, lentils, and peanuts), and grains and foods derived from them (wheat, corn, barley, couscous, brown rice, etc.). Fiber is not found in animal products.

Fiber is helpful for those trying to lose weight for several reasons. First, it adds bulk to your diet, so you feel full faster and keep feeling full longer. Foods that are high in fiber tend to be low in fat

Dr. Ian's Tip

Don't be fooled by muffins. A large muffin can contain as many as 400 calories. So while a blueberry muffin sounds healthy because of the blueberries, remember that it's packing an entire meal's worth of calories! Avoid these high-calorie foods as much as possible!

and calories, so you'll be eating much healthier if you boost the fiber in your diet. A bonus is that foods rich in fiber tend to take longer to chew. This could translate into your eating slower, getting full faster, and thus eating less overall.

Fiber is also believed to play a potential role in preventing or reducing the risk of developing cancer, diabetes, and heart disease. A high-fiber diet can help reduce colon and rectal cancer. Fiber is believed to help lower blood sugars, thus possibly reducing the need for diabetes medications and insulin injections. Several years of research have shown that a high-fiber diet could also help reduce one's risk for heart disease by lowering LDL ("bad") cholesterol. (You can find a list of fiber-rich foods on pages 207–209.)

GLYCEMIC INDEX (GI)

This has become one of those buzz phrases you hear almost every time someone uses the word "diet." Many think it's a new concept, but it has been around for more than twenty years. Yet it's only recently that scientists have gained a greater understanding of GI, which is why you've probably heard more about it and why it's getting so much coverage in the media. Glycemic index sounds complicated, but you don't need a medical degree to understand the basic principles. There have been entire books written on the glycemic index, but I'll attempt to explain the major concepts to you in a few paragraphs. Here goes.

When we consume foods that are made primarily of sugars, such as vegetables, fruits, bread, cookies, sodas, etc., the body works very hard to break down these larger sugars into their simplest, most basic form—glucose. It's critical that we break down these foods into the simple sugar glucose, because glucose is the body's greatest source of fuel. The glycemic index ranks foods based on how fast the body breaks them down into simple sugar or glucose. The faster a food is broken down into glucose, the faster and higher the levels of glucose rise in the blood. The faster your blood glucose levels rise, the stronger the signal that's sent to your pancreas to release the hormone insulin into the blood.

Insulin's primary function is to sweep up the excess sugar from the blood and bring it into the cells where it can be used right away as a source of energy, stored for future use in the form of glycogen, or stored as the dreaded fat if the body doesn't need energy at the time. It's this last function of insulin that diet experts worry about and believe might cause excessive weight gain in people who eat lots of high GI foods. The idea is to eat foods that have a lower GI, so blood glucose levels won't rise as quickly, and the body's insulin response won't be as dramatic. This would mean there's less chance for the insulin to sweep up the glucose into the cells, where it could be converted and stored as fat.

Dr. Ian's Tip

Keep a food journal. Writing down what you eat, how much you eat, and when you do your exercise is a great way to keep you on the right track. Jot down the times you feel hungry or tired or irritable just because you want that piece of chocolate. Journaling can be a great tool to keep you honest and expose the bad habits that are interfering with your weight-loss efforts. Don't look at it as a core, but as a strategy to better understand your habits and a way to make smarter decisions.

Just for the sake of comparison, glucose is randomly assigned a GI value of 100. The way the table below works is that the other foods are compared to glucose's value. The lower the GI number, the more slowly the food is broken down into glucose.

HIGH GI	LARGE GI	LOW GI
>70	56-69	<55

Here's a smaller version of the glycemic index to help you understand where some of the common foods reside. Carbohydrates are listed because it's the speed of breakdown of carbohydrates that gives us the glycemic index number.

FOOD	GLYCEMIC INDEX (GLUCOSE = 100)	SERVING SIZE	CARBOHYDRATES PER SERVING (G)
Dates, dried	103	2 oz	40
Corn flakes	81	1 cup	26
Jelly beans	78	1 oz	28
Puffed rice cakes	78	3 cakes	21
Russet potato (baked)	76	1 large	30
Doughnut	76	1 large	23
Soda crackers	74	4 crackers	17
White bread	73	1 large slice	14
Table sugar (sucrose)	68	2 teaspoons	10
Pancake	67	6" diameter	58
White rice (boiled)	64	1 cup	36
Brown rice (boiled)	55	1 cup	33

(continued)

FOOD	GLYCEMIC INDEX (GLUCOSE = 100)	SERVING SIZE	CARBOHYDRATES PER SERVING (G)
Spaghetti, white (boiled 10–15 min)	44	1 cup	40
Orange	42	1 large	11
Rye or pumpernickel bread	41	1 large slice	12
Spaghetti, white (boiled 5 min)	38	1 cup	40
Pear	38	1 large	11
Apple	38	1 large	15
All-Bran cereal	38	1 cup	23
Spaghetti, whole wheat (boiled)	37	1 cup	37
Skim milk	32	8 ounces	13
Lentils, dried (boiled)	29	1 cup	18
Kidney beans, dried (boiled)	28	1 cup	25
Pearl barley (boiled)	25	1 cup	42
Cashew nuts	22	1 ounce	9
Peanuts	14	1 ounce	6

Source: K. Foster-Powell, S. H. Holt, and J. C. Brand-Miller, "International Table of Glycemic Index and Glycemic Load Values: 2002," *American Journal of Clinical Nutrition* 76, no. 1 (2002): 5–56.

TIMING

One of my favorite expressions is, "Timing in life is everything!" That applies to a vast array of situations—including **EXTREME FAT SMASH**. The daily meal plans in the following chapters are neatly laid out for you, but when you eat these meals and snacks is as important as what you consume. Your body is a finely tuned machine that requires fuel in the form of food energy to run efficiently at peak performance. One of the biggest mistakes we make is running our body while the gas gauge is on E. That's what happens when we skip meals or leave too much time between meals. These are two bad habits that you will break with this program.

Spacing your meals approximately every 3 hours is one of the keys to your success on the **EXTREME FAT SMASH DIET** schedule. By sticking to this, you accomplish several things: (1) you never operate your machine on empty, which is when you get the lowest performance; (2) you will not have between-meal hunger pangs and cravings; (3) you will not eat oversized portions, which practically ensures overconsumption of calories and irregular insulin surges; and (4) you might be able to prevent the release of excess cortisol, a hormone that some experts believe can increase your abdominal fat.

You have to create the schedule that works best for your individual sleep and work patterns. But whether you're a long-haul truck driver or a computer programmer, set up a schedule that follows the principles of regular and convenient timing. Here's a sample schedule that you might follow during the three cycles:

6:15	Wake up
6:40	Snack #1
6:50	Begin a cardio workout session
7:20	End workout
7:40	Breakfast
11:00	Meal #2
2:00	Meal #3
4:00	Snack #2
7:00	Meal #4
8:30	Evening workout or fast walk 1 mile
9:00	Snack #3

EXERCISE

Imagine owning an expensive sports car that can top speeds of 100 mph and more in just a matter of seconds. Now imagine four flat tires on that shiny red sports car. How fast do you think that car will be able to go now? The engine is fine, the tank is full of gas, and all of the electrical components of the car are like new. But with four flat tires that sports car will move up the road slower than a 10-ton cement truck. This is exactly what it's like to diet without exercise or exercise without the proper diet. You need to have both working together to get the best results.

If you eat healthy foods and watch your portions, you will lose a certain amount of weight. But at some point your body will grow ac-

Dr. Ian's Tip

The one meal you should never skip is breakfast, yet this is the meal that most people omit. Eating something for breakfast is critical because it gives you the energy you need to start your day and it prevents you from snacking on fattening, unhealthy foods. Your body needs fuel first thing in the morning to handle the new challenges that it will face. Skipping breakfast only increases your hunger and leads to the consumption of larger meals throughout the rest of the day. Not fueling up in the morning can also slow down your metabolism. Remember the old proverb: Breakfast like a king, lunch like a prince, dinner like a pauper.

customed to your healthy eating style and hold on to any excess weight you haven't lost yet, stopping the weight loss you've been enjoying dead in its tracks. This is why exercise is critical. Remember, the sports car with the flat tires can move, but at a much slower pace than if the tires were full of air. Put four new tires on the car and it's back to ripping down the road at warp speed. Those four tires represent exercise. Add a regular schedule of physical activity and exercise to your diet program and watch the fat and pounds burn away.

Whatever you do, don't think of exercise as a chore. It's this negative attitude that leads many people to skip it and waste a valuable opportunity not only to lose weight but also to vastly improve their overall health. Exercise will definitely help you reach your weight-loss goals faster and maintain your success, but it can provide other key benefits, such as preventing heart disease and stroke, reducing your risk of diabetes, adding years to your life, dramatically increasing your chances of recovery if you're hospitalized, reducing your risk of the bone-thinning disease osteoporosis, fighting depression, lowering the risk of cancers of the colon, prostate, and uterus, as well as numerous other health rewards.

Losing weight doesn't require an expensive membership to a gym. It is true that by using the machines in the gym such as a treadmill, elliptical, or stationary bicycle, you can get the work you need to get done more efficiently and in the shortest amount of time. But there are plenty of exercises that you can do right at home or at the local high school track that can serve you just as well. It might take you a little longer to achieve the same calorie burn as what you could achieve with machines, but at the end of the day you can still hit your target.

One device that is most helpful is a pedometer, an inexpensive, small device that you can clip onto your waistband. The pedometer counts how many steps you take, so simply put it on in the morning and wear it throughout the day. Take it off during your exercise periods, then put it back on when you're done. The idea is to get you to take a certain number of steps per day during your regular routine. Each step you take burns calories. As a general guide, 6,000 steps is a reasonable target for improving your health, while 10,000 steps is approximately what you'll need to help weight loss.

Bottom line: regular exercise is one of the best things you can do not only to lose weight but also to live a longer and healthier life. Use the box below to maximize your fat burning while working out.

CARDIO FAT BURNING

Work out with your heart rate in the fat-burning zone: 60–70 percent of your maximum heart rate. Subtract your age from 220 to find your maximum heart rate. Take this number and multiply by .60—this is the minimum heart rate you should maintain while performing your physical activity. Then take your maximum heart rate and multiply it by .70—the upper range for maximal fat burning.

EXAMPLE (40-year-old person):
220 − 40 = 180 (maximum heart rate)
180 × .60 = 108 (lower limit of minimal fat-burning range)
180 × .70 = 126 (upper limit of maximal fat-burning range)

Range during exercise for maximal fat burning: 108–126 beats per minute
NOTE: THOSE WHO ARE BETTER CONDITIONED SHOULD WORK WITHIN THE RANGE OF 60–75 PERCENT OF MAXIMUM HEART RATE.

CHAPTER 3

Extreme Fat Smash Diet Instructions

I've designed this program to be simple and easy to understand. There are too many programs already out there that are just too complicated or practically require some advanced degree just to understand. So let's get down to the business of **EXTREME FAT SMASH**.

Each week on **EXTREME FAT SMASH** is called a cycle. There are 3 cycles in the entire diet. These 3 cycles equal 1 rotation. It looks something like this:

> 1 week = 1 cycle
> 3 cycles = 1 rotation

The diet is constructed so that most people will lose 12 pounds after 3 weeks (1 rotation). Notice that I said "most people." This was not by accident. Some people are going to lose a little less and some people will lose a little more. You must first decide how much you're trying to lose. Let's say you want to lose 15 pounds. This is how it might work on **EXTREME FAT SMASH**:

```
Cycle 1..........4 pounds
Cycle 2..........4 pounds
Cycle 3..........4 pounds
```

That rotation gives you a total of 12 pounds, but you're looking to lose 15. So your next step is to go through one more cycle. Go back and do *either* Cycle 1 or Cycle 2. Don't do Cycle 3, as you just finished that cycle and you must mix up the routine to prevent your body from adjusting and slowing down or stopping weight loss. Let's say you choose to do Cycle 2. Your weight-loss log could look something like this:

```
Cycle 1..........4 pounds
Cycle 2..........4 pounds
Cycle 3..........4 pounds
Cycle 4..........3 pounds
_____

total loss     15 pounds
```

You've hit your goal—now what? This is where **EXTREME FAT SMASH** differs from other diet programs. Now that you have the 15 pounds off and you're fitting into that great gown or looking dapper in the tux you haven't been able to wear in two years, it's time to keep this weight off beyond the date of your big event. This means you must go directly into MAINTENANCE. This is the phase that you will live in forever, eating in a healthy manner and exercising to stay in good condition. One big difference is that you will not be pushing yourself the way you did for your initial rotation. I'll talk about MAINTENANCE a little later.

There are many people who want to lose more than 12 or 15 pounds. How do they make use of **EXTREME FAT SMASH**? One of the beauties of this program is its flexibility, which allows you to customize the diet so that it works for you. You can do as much of a rotation as you need to hit your target, or you can do several rotations if you choose to lose even more weight. Regardless of how many rotations you finish, once you hit your goal, it's important that you go into MAINTENANCE and stay there.

If you decide to do multiple rotations, do not expect to have the same results with each rotation. You have probably lost a considerable amount of weight, which means your body is adjusting to this loss and resisting losing any more. With each successive rotation, expect to lose no more than 80–90 percent of the previous rotation's loss. Three rotations could yield a weight-loss pattern like this:

Rotation 1	12 pounds
Rotation 2	10 pounds
Rotation 3	8 pounds

Thus, completing 3 rotations could give you an approximate 30-pound weight loss in just 9 weeks. TREMENDOUS!

To reach ultimate success, it's critical that you follow **EXTREME FAT SMASH** as it is written. Because you're seeking big results in a short period of time, there's little room for error. There is a section that discusses the substitutions that you can make on the diet, but try to stick to these substitutions and don't take liberties beyond that. Each day in a cycle is carefully mapped out so that you can plan ahead what foods you'll need to eat to be successful on that day and the time you need to set aside for the exercise requirement. Having your foods lined up in advance is critical, as it will prevent you from either missing meals, reaching for the wrong foods, or desperately searching for the right foods when you're in a difficult food environment such as at a sporting event or traveling long distance. If you have an allergy to a food or you're unable to obtain a food or beverage that's on the day's meal plan, look at the substitution list and see what else you can swap in.

Do not skip meals! It's very important that you eat the four smaller meals each day. Also, don't worry about starting the first day of a cycle on a Monday. In fact, many people prefer to start the program so that the two-a-day workout periods fall on a weekend. I strongly recommend keeping the days in the order that I've written them, but if for some pressing reason you need to switch day 2 with

Dr. Ian's Tip

Don't weigh yourself every day. Your body weight normally fluctuates day to day and even several times during the day. Weighing yourself too frequently will not give you an accurate measure of whether you're losing or gaining weight. It can also drive you crazy. Use the same scale when weighing yourself and try to do it once a week at the same time and in the same clothes (or no clothes). This will give you an accurate measure of your progress or regress.

day 5, then go ahead and do that. Just make sure you fulfill the eating and exercise requirements for whatever day you're following and that you do all seven days in a cycle.

There are journal pages provided with each of the daily plans. Journaling each day is a critical part of the program. This should be a fun exercise, because it will allow you to go back to the different days and see what worked for you and what didn't. You don't need to spend a lot of time on this, just enough to record the essentials of what you ate, your exercise log, and what you might've been feeling throughout the day, whether it's hungry, more energized, little desire to eat a scheduled meal because you're still full, etc. These notes are critical: you'll be able to review them before you decide to go on to the next cycle and make any necessary changes.

In the next chapter you will learn what "dieting type" you are. This chapter will show you which track you will follow as you go through the daily plans. Depending on your dieting type, you may have to make some slight alterations to the plan, but doing this can mean the difference between reaching your goals or falling short.

MAINTENANCE

Now that you have lost weight in a healthy manner by eating right and exercising regularly, you want to keep this weight off. **EXTREME FAT SMASH DIET** is designed not only for short-term results but also long-term benefits. Why throw away all of the progress you've made by slipping into old habits and forgetting the smart choices that have brought you success? The MAINTENANCE phase will help you hold your ground, and if you're still motivated, you could lose even more weight.

When you're finished with the cycles that you want to complete, go into MAINTENANCE and stay there as long as you want. If you start gaining weight, leave MAINTENANCE and cycle back into the diet until you've lost the weight again, then return to MAINTE-NANCE. The important thing is that the method of weight loss you're using is healthy, so the results you obtain will be positive not only when it comes to the numbers on a scale but also to your overall health. Whether you suffer from high blood pressure, diabetes, or high cholesterol levels, eating healthier and exercising more effectively can help you manage your condition and in some cases help you return completely to normal.

CHAPTER 4

Which Dieting Type Are You?

The greatest thing about human beings is our uniqueness. There are no two people anywhere in the world exactly alike. Even identical twins who share the same DNA aren't exactly alike. One might be a little taller, the other might have a longer chin or larger ears. Given the fact that there are physical and personality differences even between two people who have identical DNA, what does that mean for weight loss? Given our uniqueness, no two people will lose weight the same way. Best friends could eat the same food, exercise the same amount of time, and get the same amount of sleep, yet still lose different amounts of weight at different speeds.

Every month I receive thousands of e-mails from dieters who, according to their account, have been "perfect" on my FAT SMASH DIET but are upset because a relative or friend or neighbor has lost more weight than they have in the same amount of time. Does this mean they are doing something wrong? Possibly, but not necessarily. Does it mean the diet doesn't work? Absolutely not. Does it mean the other person is working harder? Possibly, but not necessarily. The answer could be this simple: you are a particular "dieting type" that simply doesn't lose weight easily or fast because your body—for all kinds of reasons that are out of your control—fights to hold on to weight and won't let it go.

First, let's get some definitions out of the way. By "dieting type" I mean the way your body responds to dieting. I have broken the dieting response into 3 general categories: type alpha (α), type beta (β), and type gamma (γ). Here is how they break down:

TYPE α (ALPHA)

These are people whom many would consider to be lucky. They are able to "loosely" follow a diet while occasionally taking liberties by eating foods that aren't part of the program and not doing all of the required exercise. Yet they still lose a considerable amount of weight. This dieting type can go on and off diets at their leisure and get results each time they go on a diet. They might be blessed with a fast metabolism, or their body simply responds better to food changes. For reasons that are likely to be largely out of their control,

Dr. Ian's Tip

If you have an intense craving for something to the point that you can't stop thinking about it, then go ahead and treat yourself to a small amount. Let's say you're dying for some chocolate. Go ahead and have three Hershey's Kisses (approximately 75 calories). Eating a little of what you crave may prevent you from eating too much of it when the craving becomes too strong too ignore. Understand that this is a compromise, so be content with the treat but don't overdo it.

they can succeed on programs with only moderate effort. So just imagine how successful they'd be if they followed the program intensely.

TYPE β (BETA)

These people must work hard and follow the diet almost to the letter to achieve their goals. This dieting type can eat in a healthy manner and do the right exercises yet lose only a moderate amount of weight. A couple of days of not following the program guidelines and they suffer major setbacks. As a point of comparison, if the α type were to lose 6 pounds over a given period of time, the β type would lose only 4 pounds, though they worked harder and remained more loyal to the principles of the diet. Sometimes it's difficult to pinpoint why this type doesn't lose weight as easily as the alphas, but a lot of it could have to do with a slower metabolism, adverse hormonal conditions, or a body that quickly adjusts to the eating/exercise routine and thus becomes more efficient and less likely to burn calories as fast as it did at the beginning of the program. This dieting type works hard, but it can get great results.

TYPE γ (GAMMA)

These people probably consider themselves to be unlucky. They work harder than anyone else, rarely if ever stray from the program, do more than what is asked of them, yet their weight loss results tend to be modest at best. The γ types tend to fare well at the beginning of a program but quickly hit a wall, and regardless of the changes they make to bust through that wall, they remain at a standstill. Several weeks of this lack of progress, and frustration sets in. They spend a lot of time and energy trying to figure out what they're doing wrong, when really they're following the diet perfectly. Why is losing weight so difficult for the gammas? A lot of it has to do with internal physiology that they have little control over. They might suffer from an underactive thyroid (hypothyroid), be taking medications with side effects that make weight loss difficult, and/or suffer from a very slow metabolism. Over a certain period of time, if the alphas lost 6 pounds, and the betas lost 4 pounds, then the gammas might lose only 2 pounds. The γ type is the one most likely to get frustrated, give up on a diet, then pick up another diet hoping it will be the answer.

These are general categories that most people belong to. Of course, some people share traits from all three types, but the idea is to find which dieting type fits you best, because this classification will be important in the way you attack **EXTREME FAT SMASH**. While the key to success for *everyone* is following the program as closely as possible and remaining dedicated and focused, there are some minor alterations/enhancements that should be made to get the best results possible depending on your body type. The reason for helping you identify your dieting type is not for you to complain or be envious of someone who belongs to another type. It's so you'll know what you're working with before beginning the program. It's analogous to a team about to begin a soccer game. If you know your team doesn't have enough speed to match the other players or your goalie isn't as quick and responsive as your opponent's, then you have to adjust your strategy accordingly before kickoff. This is also true for your dieting type. Knowing what advantages and disadvantages you come to a diet with will help you take a good dieting program and make it even better.

ALTERATIONS AND ENHANCEMENTS

TYPE α

You have the fewest excuses. The biggest thing standing in the way of total success is YOU! It's like the child with a superior IQ who has the aptitude to excel in the classroom, but because he applies himself only on a part-time basis, his performance is less than it could be and he gets the same results as other children who are not as "naturally gifted." You have an excellent chance to be unbelievably successful on **EXTREME FAT SMASH**. Your major task is to avoid falling into a zone of complacency because you know that regardless of what you do, you're still going to lose something. Your biggest task is to keep disciplined and stay determined to give it your all through each cycle of the diet you choose to follow. You have been blessed with a dieting type and physiology to excel on this program. Don't throw away your blessings and be satisfied with underachieving.

TYPE β

You will be making some modest tweaks to the daily plans as laid out in the next chapter. You need to continuously keep your body guessing so that it doesn't grow accustomed to your routine or the weight that you've already lost. This means cutting back on your portions some days and increasing your exercise on others. Of all the types, you will benefit most from remaining extremely faithful to the exercise portion, because this will be your greatest chance of burning the most calories in the shortest amount of time. There's no question that you can reach goals, but your ultimate weight loss will be a matter of how creative you are and how much you're willing to change things even when you're doing what's right. What does that mean? If the daily plan says that you can eat 1 cup of brown rice at a meal, will you be willing to eat only a ½ cup? If the cycle instructions say that you can have two glasses of wine for the week, are you willing to give back a glass and only have one? These small changes will enhance your results and bring you a greater chance of success.

TYPE γ

This is my favorite group. The odds are stacked against the gammas relative to the other two types, and it would be so easy for you to give in to frustration and quit. But this is where your heart and soul come into play. *You are not a quitter!* You have an iron resolve to see this program through to the end and not succumb to the disappointments that may dot your path to success. Because your body tends to work against you, or your medications are making it difficult to lose weight, you must approach this program methodically. Never focus beyond today. You must work like a mechanic, pulling things apart, keeping track of the parts, then putting them back together. Your biggest challenge will be remaining positive regardless of the

Dr. Ian's Tip

If you're having trouble keeping your portions under control, try this: instead of a large dinner plate, serve your meal on a smaller salad plate and leave a one-inch perimeter around the food—always make sure you can see plenty of plate when you serve anything except salad! Don't go back for seconds. Instead, grab a piece of fruit or low-fat dessert if you're still hungry.

hurdles you face or the results you obtain. But your triumph at the end of the journey will be so much greater because of all the adversity you faced. On each daily plan, find your tweak notes and consider them the great equalizers that will help you be just as successful as the alphas and betas. You will be asked to do some things differently, but it's important from a psychological perspective that you look at these instructions as rewards and not penalties. You *can* get this done and it will be your determination that ultimately carries you across the finish line.

CHAPTER 5

Metabolism: Our Internal Engine

Dieting and metabolism seem to be joined at the hip. Whether in advertisements, magazines, or conversations around the office water cooler, when someone talks about dieting, she inevitably talks about metabolism. But what is metabolism? Many people have some idea, but there tend to be many misperceptions mixed in with the facts. By the time you finish this chapter, I want you to have a basic understanding of what is meant by metabolism and why it can be important in your efforts to lose weight.

WHAT IS IT?

Every living thing has a metabolism. We are all born with it, and regardless of whether it's fast or slow, it's working every second of our lives—even when we're sleeping. Metabolism is the process that converts the fuel that's in the food we eat into the energy we need to do everything we do, whether it's getting up from a chair, typing on a computer, watching TV, running five miles, or reading this sentence. There are thousands of small reactions occurring at the same time within your body to burn fuel so that you can live and perform a variety of functions. This burning of fuel is the burning of calories. So whether you're consuming a big slice of pizza, a bowl of oatmeal, or a garden salad, each has a certain number of calories (fuel), and the body burns these calories to get the energy it needs to perform the functions you want to carry out. Put another way, your metabolism is the rate at which your body burns calories to sustain life. I like to think of metabolism as a car's engine transplanted into your body. An engine makes the car move. The engine can operate only if it has fuel. The better the fuel, the better the engine runs. The bigger the engine, the more fuel it burns. Even when your car is sitting idle, it's using fuel. When it's speeding down the road, it uses even more fuel. Your metabolism works the same way. This is also why it's important to eat smaller meals throughout the day and not wait until you're extremely hungry, then sit down for one big meal. Just like a car that stops in the pit to be refueled and checked periodically for peak performance, your body needs steady and reliable nourishment to keep your energy levels high and your metabolism speeding along. Remember this when you're eating and exercising or deciding to sit idle on the couch.

Dr. Ian's Tip

Schedule your exercise. Enough with the excuses about not having time to exercise. Treat exercise just like you do an important business meeting or a hair appointment. Mark the time on your calendar or in your BlackBerry. Giving exercise a regular appointment time will help you not only remember that it's time to get moving, but also help make it a necessary priority.

WHAT AFFECTS YOUR METABOLISM

Several things—both internal and external—can have an effect on your metabolism. Some things will speed it up while others can slow it down. I will briefly discuss the things that have the biggest impact on your metabolism. Understanding this list will help you make smart decisions in your weight-loss journey.

MUSCLE TISSUE

Muscle has a big impact on your metabolic rate. In general, the more muscle you have, the higher your metabolic rate. Muscle is the body's biggest calorie burner whether you're exercising or resting.

MEAL FREQUENCY

Eating is another function that requires energy. So while you're consuming food full of calories, you also need to burn other calories to actually carry out the tasks of eating and digestion. The longer you wait between meals, the less eating and digesting that are going on, the more your metabolism slows down.

ACTIVITY LEVEL

How active you are can greatly impact the speed of your metabolism. Whether it's working out in a gym, walking in your neighborhood, or just running around doing errands, physical activities require a great deal of energy, and that increases your metabolic rate, which in turn burns calories.

HYDRATION

Seventy to seventy-five percent of your body weight is water. That means that most of your bodily functions are taking place in water.

Dr. Ian's Tip

Have you ever wondered how many calories you might be burning just by living? According to the Rule of 10, the body burns about 10 calories per pound of body weight to meet basic energy needs. Let's say you weigh 160 pounds. You would burn about 1,600 calories (160×10 calories per pound) per day for your basal metabolism (energy your body burns just to exist). These 1,600 calories represent only 60 percent of the total calories you need for basic energy needs. This means that over the course of the day you will burn 2,666 calories (1,600=60 percent of 2,666) just to exist. Add in your exercise and you could be burning well over 3,000 calories a day. To lose a pound you need to burn off 3,500 excess calories *above* what it takes to maintain your weight.

If you're not hydrated properly with water and other fluids, then all of your systems could slow down, including metabolism.

GENETICS

Our metabolic rate is largely out of our control because it tends to be something that we're born with, just as we're born to be a certain height or to have a certain eye color. The DNA we inherit from our parents typically determines our metabolic fate. Some are destined to have a fast metabolism, while others have one that runs at a slower rate. There are things we can do to make some changes to our metabolic rate, but for most of us the big decision was made before we were even born.

AGING

Many people believe that simply getting older causes the metabolism to slow. There's a kernel of truth in this, but I don't buy it as an excuse for weight gain. The real issue with aging is that we tend to be less active and as a result we lose our muscle mass. Participating in less physical activity and losing your muscle can slow your metabolism.

HORMONES

Several hormones can affect metabolism to varying degrees. These include thyroid, growth, estrogen, and testosterone. Your body's ability to produce the adequate amount of properly functioning hormones can have a positive or negative effect on your metabolism.

REVVING UP YOUR ENGINE

Now that you understand how important your metabolism is in burning calories and helping you lose weight, you can understand why one of the most commonly asked dieting questions is: how can I speed up my metabolism? If you were to go on the Internet, flip through fitness magazines, or watch those late-night infomercials, you would undoubtedly come across several sales pitches about the latest and greatest supplement or method to speed up your metabolism. The unfortunate truth is that most of these claims are completely inaccurate and downright dishonest. Remember, weight loss is a multibillion-dollar industry, which means there are a lot of people who see their fortunes in your eagerness to lose weight.

Dr. Ian's Tip

Bookend your workouts. When you exercise, you speed up your metabolism, and this effect can last up to several hours depending on the intensity and length of your workout. This elevation in metabolism means that after you've finished your exercise, you're still burning calories. So why not take advantage of this prolonged effect by bookending your workouts? Work out in the morning, then do another workout in the late afternoon or evening. You'll have instant elevated metabolism through a good portion of the day.

The simple truth is that you can do some things to speed up your metabolism, but you cannot speed up your metabolism so much that the "fat just melts away," as many advertising slogans would have you believe. But if there are some things you can do to turn up your calorie burner, then why not give them a try? The most important thing is to understand that increasing your metabolism is only one component of weight loss. You need to do the whole package of **EXTREME FAT SMASH** for total success.

BUILD LEAN MUSCLE MASS

The body's percentage of lean muscle mass is believed to have the biggest impact on metabolism. You don't have to become a body-builder in order to take advantage of this metabolic-boosting strategy. You should begin a program of resistance exercises using resistance bands or lifting light free weights. The idea is to tone your muscles and make them nice and firm. Maintaining muscles burns a lot of calories, so the more muscle you have, the more calories you'll burn. And even while resting, your muscles are burning more calories. A note of caution: if you have never been trained in proper weight-lifting techniques, get some supervision from a professional before you begin following a program on your own.

REGULAR EATING SCHEDULE

Believe it or not, one of the easiest ways to improve your metabolism might be as simple as eating your meals on a regular schedule. One of the biggest mistakes people make is skipping meals. Too many people think that by skipping meals they'll lose weight faster because they're eating less. The reality is much different. The process of eating can actually increase your metabolism; if you don't eat, your metabolism can slow down. When you skip meals, your body switches its metabolism into "starvation mode," because it doesn't know if or when it will get more food again. When this happens, your body is likely to store more calories as fat rather than break down the fat cells and use the previously stored energy. When your body goes into starvation mode, it's like a car whose battery has died. To get the car going again, it needs a jump start. You can jump-start your metabolism by resuming a regular schedule of eating smaller meals. This will not only keep your metabolism revving, it also will keep your blood sugar and insulin levels steady, which can be critical in weight loss.

Over the course of the day, you should try to eat something every three hours. I'm not suggesting that you eat large meals, but instead small, portion-controlled meals that will keep your energy levels up and prevent you from going long periods of time feeling hungry. If you're unable to have a complete meal, have a snack that will keep you going until the next meal.

Dr. Ian's Tip

Try not to eat your meals on the run. The faster you eat, the more you eat, because you don't give your stomach and brain enough time to register that you are full. This causes you to eat past your satiety point. Eat slowly and think about how much you're enjoying the flavor and texture of your food. Eating should be a pleasurable experience.

STAY HYDRATED

Your mother was right: water is good for you. Lack of water can slow your metabolic rate just the way a lack of food can. Water is the body's most important nutrient, and without it your body temperature can drop and cause you to store fat. Research has shown that not consuming enough water can reduce your body's ability to burn calories by 2 percent each day. Drink at least 6 glasses of water each day. Other good sources of hydration are the sports-type drinks. You should limit the amount of caffeinated beverages you drink, such as soda, coffee, and tea, as your body absorbs only approximately half of the liquid in them.

REDUCE STRESS

"Don't worry, be happy" is more than just a memorable line in a song. It should be a guide for most of us to follow when it comes to reducing our stress and increasing our relaxation. Research is continuously being published that demonstrates how stress can have a biological impact on our ability to function. Whether you work in a difficult environment or you're constantly arguing with your next-door neighbor, continual stress can take a toll on your body in ways you don't even see. Stress leads to a hormonal firestorm in your body that can cause all kinds of problems, including elevating the levels of stress hormones, which ultimately slow your metabolism and increase your appetite at the same time. There are plenty of things you can do to reduce stress. If you can't totally eliminate the major stress triggers from your life, try some simple techniques such as 10 minutes of meditation a day, a daily 15-minute peaceful walk, listening to soothing music, reading a book, or simply sitting on a park bench and doing nothing. Figure out what relaxes you and then dedicate some time every day to at least one stress-relieving activity.

GET MOVING

If I could prescribe only one thing to improve not only your metabolism but also your overall health, it would be an increase in physical activity. Movement—whether it's climbing a couple of flights of stairs or walking/running on a treadmill in the gym—dramatically increases your body's energy needs, which must be fueled. This fuel will be calories, and this increased calorie burning is the definition of a speeded-up metabolism. Splitting up your exercise into two or more sessions during the day is a smart way to speed up your metabolism while barely noticing the effort.

INCREASE THE PROTEIN

Protein-rich foods can help boost your metabolism, because protein burns more energy during digestion than any other macronutrient. Foods that are high in protein include chicken, beans, lentils, fish, chickpeas, eggs, lean cuts of beef, cottage cheese, and turkey. It's generally recommended that most people consume approximately 80 grams of protein per day. To see how much protein you're con-

Dr. Ian's Tip

Eat as many meals as possible sitting down without being distracted. Don't eat in front of the TV or computer; instead sit down with friends or family and enjoy the meal as well as the company. Eating while doing something else tends to cause you to eat large portions and not truly enjoy the food or company with whom you're sharing the meal. People who work in offices should try to avoid eating at their desks. It's important to clear your mind and change your environment. If you are eating alone, try reading a good book, newspaper, or magazine.

suming, look at the nutrition label on the packaging. There is, however, a caveat you need to be mindful of while trying to boost your metabolism. Too much protein can also lead to problems, such as kidney damage, calcium depletion, and ketosis where you could be at risk for heart disease and high blood pressure. So you need to make sure that you don't overdo protein.

GO TO BED

New research has given us better insight into the effect of sleep on our metabolism and weight-loss efforts. Simply put, those who don't sleep enough tend to have a more difficult time losing weight. This is partly attributed to stress hormones. When you don't sleep enough, your body produces more stress hormones, which slows your metabolism and increases production of hormones that affect your appetite. Not everyone needs the same amount of sleep. The traditional 8 hours is a safe goal, but some people require less and some require more. You have to figure out the amount you need so that you wake up in the morning feeling completely rested and energized. Try going to bed an entire week without setting an alarm clock and see how many hours you sleep naturally, waking up when your body says it's had enough rest. That could give you some idea of how many hours of sleep you actually need.

CHAPTER 6

Cycle 1

This is the moment that you've been waiting for, the time to take your first steps toward changing your life, getting rid of that stubborn extra weight, and building a NEW YOU! Read each day's plan very carefully and make sure you've studied it far enough in advance to have the foods you need on hand and the time to do your exercise lined up. There is a long list of snacks that you're encouraged to have on the program. You can find this snack list on pages 130–133. These snacks are not meals, so do not use them that way. The meals that you'll be eating are likely to be smaller than you're accustomed to, and that's the way I've designed it. There will be enough that you will be full, not so much that you'll be stuffed. If you're still feeling hungry after your meal, wait an hour, then enjoy one of the snacks.

Pay close attention to the exercise. The amount that you're asked to do each day has been chosen carefully to match what you're eating that day and your current stage in the program. You now have what you need to succeed. Go SMASH it!

CYCLE 1 GUIDELINES

PLEASE READ CAREFULLY

- You're allowed up to 2 snacks each day. The snacks must be 100 calories or less. You don't have to eat snacks; it's up to you. But if you do, follow the guidelines. Remember, snacks are a great way to keep your body properly fueled throughout the day so that you can continue to reach peak performance.
- You can have 3 tablespoons of low-fat or fat-free salad dressing a day.
- You can drink up to 2 cans of diet soda per day, but remember that less is more.
- You can drink up to 1 cup of low-fat, fat-free, or soy milk per day, whether it's in your cereal or by itself. The milk you use in your protein shake or smoothie doesn't count against this 1 cup total.
- Drink as much plain water as you like and at any time of the day. I recommend that you drink at least 6 cups per day.
- You're allowed to have 1 SMALL cup (8 ounces) of coffee and 1 SMALL cup of tea each day.
- You're allowed to have two 6-ounce glasses of wine for the entire week.
- 1 vegetable serving is roughly the size of a small fist.
- You can have condiments with your meals. Choose 2 items below per meal, or break them up over several meals:

    Mustard: 1 teaspoon

    Mayo: 1 teaspoon

    Ketchup: 1 teaspoon

    Relish: 1 teaspoon

    Salsa: ¼ cup

    Hot sauce: 2 tablespoons

    Soy sauce: 2 tablespoons

- You're allowed to have 6-ounce servings of yogurt where specified in the meal plan, but it should be low-fat or fat-free and NOT the kind with the fruit on the bottom.
- Your vegetables can be steamed, grilled, boiled, or raw. You can also cook them with a little oil or butter spray.
- NO bread, white rice, white potato, baked beans, banana, pineapple, or watermelon during this cycle.
- NO cottage cheese or peanut butter during this cycle.
- All protein shakes and fruit smoothies should be less than 200 calories.
- Salt is allowed, but no more than 1 teaspoon per day.
- Turkey and chicken are to be baked, roasted, boiled, or grilled and eaten without the skin.
- Add some flavor to your veggies or rice by adding 1–2 tablespoons of soy sauce.
- For your fruits, load up on berries. They're full of vitamins and cancer-fighting antioxidants. Apples, oranges, and pears are full of healthy fiber.
- If your stomach is rumbling between meals, try chewing a stick of sugarless gum. You can have unlimited carrots and celery between meals. This can help carry you until your next meal.
- The exercise program is critical to your success. You MUST do the exercise for optimal results. The daily required amounts are the *minimum* that you must do. If you want to do more, that's GREAT! Consider these extra minutes bonus dollars. The more you do, the more bonus dollars you collect!
- When you have a "two-a-day," which means two different exercise periods in a day, try to separate them by at least 6 hours for maximum effectiveness. This will help your metabolism stay elevated for a greater part of the day.
- On REST DAYS, you are not required to do any of the regi-

mented exercises. However, stay active by walking around and keeping busy. Remember, you can still do exercise on rest days. The calories you burn will be like collecting bonus dollars. What would it hurt to do 25 minutes of exercise even on a rest day? This brings you closer to your goal!

Day 1

MEALS

BREAKFAST

2 egg whites or ½ cup of Egg Beaters or 1 whole egg (cooked with light oil or butter spray)

1 piece of fruit (no banana/watermelon/pineapple) **OR** ½ cup of freshly squeezed fruit or tomato juice

MEAL #2

1 cup of sliced fresh fruit (no banana/watermelon/pineapple). You might want to mix it for a variety of taste. You can find fresh fruit cups premade at the grocery store.

MEAL #3

1 small salad (veggies only) with 3 tablespoons of low-fat or fat-free dressing

MEAL #4

½ cup of beans, lentils, or chickpeas

2 servings of vegetables

γ: *1 serving of vegetables*

EXERCISE

55 minutes of cardio. Try doing at least 2 different exercises to comprise the 55 minutes. For example, 25 minutes fast walking/running on the treadmill and 30 minutes on the stationary bicycle. Make sure you stay within your fat-burning heart range.

β: *60 minutes of cardio*

γ: *65 minutes of cardio*

Dr. Ian's Tip

Bagels are not your friends. If there's one thing you should either drastically reduce in your diet or cut out altogether, it's bagels. They look innocent enough, but some bagels contain as many as 350 calories. Supersize bagels can have up to 600 calories or more. And that's without the butter, cream cheese, or jam. Stay away from bagels and use the calories for something that packs more useful nutrients and keeps you full longer.

Dr. Ian's Tip

Go to the grocery store with a shopping list. This will help you be better organized to purchase only those foods that you need to stick with your eating plan. A prepared list will also help prevent you from impulsively throwing extra foods in your cart that are not on the list and full of unnecessary calories.

Day 1 Journal Entry

BREAKFAST

Time _____

Foods _____

MEAL #2

Time _____

Foods _____

MEAL #3

Time _____

Foods _____

MEAL #4

Time _____

Foods _____

SNACKS

Time _____   Time _____   Time _____

Type and quantity _____

_____

EXERCISE

Time _____   Time _____

Types and duration _____

_____

_____

Notes _____

_____

_____

Day 2

MEALS

BREAKFAST

6 ounces of low-fat/fat-free yogurt

1 piece of fruit OR 1 cup of freshly squeezed fruit or vegetable juice

MEAL #2

1 small salad with 3 tablespoons of low-fat or fat-free dressing

1 cup of freshly squeezed fruit or vegetable juice (if you had this for breakfast, then a piece of fruit)

MEAL #3

4 ounces of fish, chicken (no skin), turkey, or lean sirloin

½ cup of beans, chickpeas, or lentils (canned or boiled in water or broth)

MEAL #4

1 cup of boiled brown rice or dirty rice

2 servings of vegetables (raw, steamed, grilled, boiled, or sautéed—this applies to all veggies)

β: ½ *cup of brown rice*

γ: ½ *cup of brown rice*

EXERCISE

35 minutes of cardio in the morning

30 minutes of cardio in the afternoon or evening (try to do a different cardio routine, if possible)

β: 40 *minutes in the morning, 30 minutes in the afternoon or evening*

γ: 45 *minutes in the morning, 40 minutes in the afternoon or evening*

Dr. Ian's Tip

Increase your consumption of fiber-rich foods (fruits, vegetables, and whole grains). These foods tend to be low in fat and calories. Fiber adds bulk to your diet, making you feel fuller faster and longer. The good thing about fiber is that it can't be digested, so it doesn't add any calories to your diet. High-fiber diets may also help reduce cancer risk and lower your risk of heart disease. Foods high in fiber include pears and apples with skin, strawberries, oranges, brussels sprouts, lentils, beans, bran cereals, oatmeal, and peanuts. (For more complete list, see Fiber chart on pages 207–209.)

Dr. Ian's Tip

Start slow. Beginners often try to do too much too fast. This common mistake unfortunately often leads to injury and discouragement. Getting in shape is not a race; it's a *process*. Steady progress is much better than trying to go for the gusto right at the beginning. Every couple of weeks, step up your workout by 10 percent. If you have been walking on the treadmill for 30 minutes per session, kick it up to 33 minutes. If you've been riding a bicycle for 1 mile per session, increase it to 1.1 miles. As you become more experienced and better conditioned, you can increase the intensity and length of your workout.

Day 2 Journal Entry

BREAKFAST

Time _____

Foods _____

MEAL #2

Time _____

Foods _____

MEAL #3

Time _____

Foods _____

MEAL #4

Time _____

Foods _____

SNACKS

Time _____   Time _____   Time _____

Type and quantity _____

_____

EXERCISE

Time _____   Time _____

Types and duration _____

_____

_____

Notes _____

_____

_____

Day 3

MEALS

BREAKFAST

1 cup of cooked oatmeal (if you use instant or flavored, 1 packet). Optional: sliced fruit/berries, ½ teaspoon of sugar, 1 teaspoon of sugar substitute, or ½ pat of butter

1 cup of freshly squeezed fruit or veggie juice **OR** 1 piece of fruit

MEAL #2

1 small fruit smoothie (no added sweeteners, must be less than 200 calories)

OR

1 small whey protein shake (200 calories or less; if using milk instead of water, use low-fat or skim milk, 1 cup or less)

MEAL #3

1 cup of cooked beans, chickpeas, or lentils (baked beans not allowed during this cycle)

1 cup of cooked brown rice

1 serving of vegetables

β: *½ cup of brown rice*

no vegetables

γ: *½ cup of brown rice*

½ cup of cooked beans, chickpeas, or lentils

no vegetables

MEAL #4

4 ounces of fish, chicken, turkey, or lean sirloin (4 ounces is
roughly the size of a deck of cards)

½ large baked sweet potato

2 servings of vegetables

β: *1 serving of vegetables*

γ: *1 serving of vegetables*

EXERCISE

55 minutes of cardio. If you want to break these 55 minutes into
smaller segments, that's fine. The entire exercise time should
have you within your fat-burning heart range.

β: *60 minutes of cardio*

γ: *65 minutes of cardio*

Dr. Ian's Tip

Use mustard instead of mayonnaise. A tablespoon of mayo contains approximately 100 calories. An equal amount of yellow mustard contains only 10 calories. Your mustard choice can make a difference also. Brown, Dijon, and honey mustards contain more calories than yellow mustard, but still many fewer than mayo.

Dr. Ian's Tip

If you typically drink regular soda, switch to diet soda and watch the number on the scale gradually decrease. Let's say that you drink one 12-ounce can of regular soda a day. If you continue to do everything as you normally do and simply switch to diet soda, you could lose approximately 16 pounds in one year. Small changes can make a big difference!

Day 3 Journal Entry

BREAKFAST

Time _____

Foods _____

MEAL #2

Time _____

Foods _____

MEAL #3

Time _____

Foods _____

MEAL #4

Time _____

Foods _____

SNACKS

Time _____ Time _____ Time _____

Type and quantity _____

_____

EXERCISE

Time _____ Time _____

Types and duration _____

_____

_____

Notes _____

_____

_____

Day 4

MEALS

BREAKFAST

6 ounces of plain or low-fat yogurt

1 piece of fruit OR ½ cup of berries (no watermelon or pineapple)

MEAL #2

1 small fresh fruit smoothie (<200 calories)

OR

1 small whey protein shake (<200 calories)

MEAL #3

1 large vegetable salad with the white of 1 hard-boiled egg

MEAL #4

1 small veggie, soy, or tofu burger (e.g., Boca or Morning Star), 1 teaspoon of ketchup or mustard allowed, but no bread

1 cup of boiled brown rice or dirty rice

γ: *½ cup of cooked brown rice*

EXERCISE

REST DAY

β: *40 minutes of cardio*

γ: *50 minutes of cardio*

Dr. Ian's Tip

Get a buddy. Exercising can be so much more productive when you have a regular partner who's doing it with you. A partner can push you when you start taking it easy and can also be a good source of friendly competition, helping you reach your goals while having some fun doing it. Workout buddies can also be a physical help, providing assistance if you need help lifting weights. Working out with someone else can also help the time go by much faster.

Day 4 Journal Entry

BREAKFAST

Time _____

Foods _____

MEAL #2

Time _____

Foods _____

MEAL #3

Time _____

Foods _____

MEAL #4

Time _____

Foods _____

SNACKS

Time _____   Time _____   Time _____

Type and quantity _____

_____

EXERCISE

Time _____   Time _____

Types and duration _____

_____

_____

Notes _____

_____

_____

Day 5

MEALS

BREAKFAST

1 egg white omelet with veggies (use 2 egg whites or ½ cup of Egg Beaters; if desired, cook with a small amount of olive oil or butter spray)

1 piece of fruit OR ½ cup of berries (no watermelon or pineapple)

MEAL #2

1 small salad

1 cup of freshly squeezed fruit or vegetable juice

MEAL #3

4 ounces of fish, chicken, turkey, or lean sirloin

1 cup of cooked beans, chickpeas, or lentils

β: ½ cup of cooked beans

γ: ½ cup of cooked beans

MEAL #4

2 servings of vegetables

1 cup of boiled brown or dirty rice

γ: ½ cup of boiled rice

EXERCISE

30 minutes of cardio in the morning

30 minutes of cardio in the afternoon or evening

β: 35 minutes in the morning, 35 minutes in the afternoon or evening

γ: 40 minutes in the morning, 40 minutes in the afternoon or evening

Day 5 Journal Entry

BREAKFAST

Time _____

Foods _____

MEAL #2

Time _____

Foods _____

MEAL #3

Time _____

Foods _____

MEAL #4

Time _____

Foods _____

SNACKS

Time _____   Time _____   Time _____

Type and quantity _____

_____

EXERCISE

Time _____   Time _____

Types and duration _____

_____

_____

Notes _____

_____

_____

Day 6

MEALS

BREAKFAST

1 egg white omelet with veggies (use 2 egg whites or ½ cup of Egg Beaters; you can use a small amount of olive oil or butter spray for cooking)

OR

1 cup of oatmeal (if you use instant or flavored, 1 packet)

1 cup of freshly squeezed fruit or vegetable juice

β: *½ cup of oatmeal*

γ: *½ cup of oatmeal*

MEAL #2

1 small fresh fruit smoothie (<200 calories)

OR

1 small whey protein shake (<200 calories)

MEAL #3

4 ounces of chicken, fish, turkey, or lean sirloin

1 serving of vegetables

½ cup of brown or dirty rice

β: *no rice*

γ: *no rice*

MEAL #4

2 servings of vegetables

½ cup of brown or dirty rice

EXERCISE

55 minutes of cardio

β: *60 minutes of cardio*

γ: *65 minutes of cardio*

Dr. Ian's Tip

Eat before the party. Lots of high-calorie temptations await you at parties. Avoid the seduction of those fattening foods by eating a small meal beforehand. When you get to the party, not only will you be less hungry, but if you still have the urge to eat, you can snack on the healthier foods and avoid those that are guaranteed to add inches to your waist. This strategy holds particularly true for those holiday bashes.

Day 6 Journal Entry

BREAKFAST

Time _____

Foods_____

MEAL #2

Time _____

Foods_____

MEAL #3

Time _____

Foods_____

MEAL #4

Time _____

Foods_____

SNACKS

Time _____   Time _____   Time _____

Type and quantity _____

_____

EXERCISE

Time _____   Time _____

Types and duration _____

_____

_____

Notes _____

_____

_____

Day 7

MEALS

BREAKFAST

6 ounces of plain, low-fat yogurt (with sliced fresh fruit or berries)

1 piece of fruit OR ½ cup of berries (no watermelon or pineapple)

MEAL #2

1 small salad (optional: 1 egg white)

½ cup of mixed sliced fruit

β: *no fruit*

γ: *no fruit*

MEAL #3

1 veggie, soy, or tofu burger (Boca or Morning Star), 1 teaspoon of ketchup or mustard, if desired

½ cup of cooked beans, chickpeas, or lentils

γ: *no beans, chickpeas, or lentils*

MEAL #4

4 ounces of fish, chicken, turkey, or lean sirloin

2 servings of vegetables

β: *1 serving of vegetables*

γ: *1 serving of vegetables*

EXERCISE

35 minutes of cardio in the morning

35 minutes of cardio in the afternoon or evening

β: *40 minutes in the morning, 40 minutes in the afternoon or evening*

γ: *45 minutes in the morning, 45 minutes in the afternoon or evening*

Dr. Ian's Tip

Weaning is a good thing. If you drink lots of coffee each day, then it's time to think about cutting back on some of that java. Some people can stop cold turkey without any side effects, while others might suffer from withdrawal headaches and mood swings. If you fall into the latter category, slowly wean yourself off the coffee. Try to reduce your daily intake by half every three weeks until you are comfortable with the amount you're drinking. Try not to exceed more than 1 cup a day.

Day 7 Journal Entry

BREAKFAST

Time _____

Foods _____

MEAL #2

Time _____

Foods _____

MEAL #3

Time _____

Foods _____

MEAL #4

Time _____

Foods _____

SNACKS

Time _____   Time _____   Time _____

Type and quantity _____

_____

EXERCISE

Time _____   Time _____

Types and duration _____

_____

_____

Notes _____

_____

_____

SUBSTITUTIONS

Below you'll find some convenient substitutions that you can make for certain items in the meal plans. Use this list as a guide for all of the cycles. The purpose of this is to give you some flexibility when preparing your meals and help you increase the variety in your foods so that you don't get bored eating the same things.

- You can always substitute 6 ounces of plain or low-fat yogurt and a piece of fruit for whatever is listed as the day's breakfast items.
- 2 egg whites = ½ cup of Egg Beaters = 1 whole egg.
- 1 cup of brown rice = 1 cup of wheat berries = ¼ cup of quinoa = 1 cup of wild rice = 1 cup of dirty rice = 1 cup of basmati rice = 1 cup of kasha = ½ cup of pearl barley
- ½ cup of fresh juice can replace a piece of fruit, and vice versa.
- Veggie burgers can be replaced by soy, tofu, or turkey burgers.
- If you can't get freshly squeezed fruit juice, you can substitute juices that say on the label "not from concentrate." Don't drink products that say "juice drink" or "juice blend," as they are full of additives and calories.
- If you can't get freshly squeezed tomato juice, you can substitute something like V8 juice, but choose the 100 percent vegetable juice product.
- 1 cup of oatmeal = 1 cup of farina = 1 cup of Cream of Wheat = ¾ cup of grits. Remember, these are the amounts after the food has been cooked.
- 1 protein shake = 1 smoothie = 1 low-fat milk shake (they all should be less than 200 calories).

CHAPTER 7

Cycle 2

CONGRATULATIONS! You have completed the first cycle of the program and now your body is primed to tackle Cycle 2. Your body is in a weight-losing mode right now, and we'll capitalize on that and keep the momentum going. For many, Cycle 1 is the most difficult part of the program because it requires you to get organized with your schedule and adhere to an eating regimen very different from your norm. But now the kinks are all worked out, and you are prepared both physically and mentally for this new cycle. Oh, by the way, wasn't it awesome to wake up this morning and see how much weight you lost in just 7 days? To think that you lost that weight naturally and in a healthy way. And you got to eat and not be hungry all day!

If the weight loss you achieved in Cycle 1 is your goal, then DOUBLE CONGRATULATIONS to you. Your next step is to turn to the MAINTENANCE chapter and read what to do next. You've gotten the weight off and with MAINTENANCE you'll keep it off. But for those who still have more distance to travel on their journey, more fat to SMASH, not to worry. This new cycle will keep you on track. Please remember the basic principles of this diet. YOU have a goal to lose a significant amount of weight in a short period of time. YOU set this goal. YOU made the commitment before starting the program to work EXTREMELY hard and remain dedicated. YOU are the one who will enjoy the delicious fruits of your labor. YOU will not fail!

Make sure you read the guidelines before starting this cycle. These guidelines will help fill in some of the gaps and provide important information about many of the new foods and behaviors allowed on this cycle.

CYCLE 2 GUIDELINES

PLEASE READ CAREFULLY

- You're allowed up to 2 snacks each day. The snacks must be 100 calories or less. You don't have to eat snacks; it's up to you. But if you do, follow the guidelines. Remember, snacks are a great way to keep your body properly fueled throughout the day so that you can continue to reach peak performance.
- You can have 3 tablespoons of low-fat or fat-free salad dressing a day.
- You can drink up to 2 cans of diet soda per day, but remember that less is more.
- You can drink up to ½ cup of lemon juice per day.
- You can drink up to 1 cup of low-fat, fat-free, skim, or soy milk per day, whether it's in your cereal or by itself. The milk you use in your protein shake or smoothie doesn't count against this 1 cup total.
- Drink as much plain water as you like and at any time of the day. I recommend that you drink at least 6 cups per day.
- You're allowed to have 1 SMALL cup (8 ounces) of coffee and 1 SMALL cup of tea each day.
- You're allowed to have two 6-ounce glasses of wine for the entire week. You're allowed to have two 12-ounce bottles or cans of beer this week. Try to drink lite beer. You're also allowed to have one

mixed drink this week. Remember, the less alcohol you drink, the more room you'll have for other, more important calories.

- You're allowed to have 6-ounce servings of yogurt, but it should be low-fat or fat-free and NOT the kind with the fruit on the bottom.
- 1 vegetable serving is roughly the size of a small fist.
- Your vegetables can be steamed, grilled, boiled, or raw. You can also cook them with a little oil or butter spray.
- 4 ounces is roughly the size of a deck of cards.
- All protein shakes and fruit smoothies should be less than 200 calories.
- Salt is allowed, but try to eat no more than 1 teaspoon per day.
- Turkey and chicken are to be baked, roasted, boiled, or grilled and eaten without the skin.
- Add some flavor to your veggies or rice by adding 1–2 tablespoons of soy sauce.
- For your fruits, load up on berries. They're full of vitamins and cancer-fighting antioxidants. Apples, oranges, and pears are full of healthy fiber.
- If your stomach is rumbling between meals, try chewing a stick of sugarless gum. You can have unlimited carrots and celery between meals. This can help carry you until your next meal.
- You can have 3 tablespoons of low-fat cottage cheese per day.
- You can have 1 tablespoon of peanut butter per day.
- With your cereals, you're allowed sliced fruit/berries, ½ teaspoon of sugar, 1 teaspoon of sugar substitute. If you're eating hot cereal, you can have ½ pat of butter.
- You can use small amounts of olive oil or butter spray when cooking.
- With your protein shakes, if you're using milk instead of water, use low-fat, skim, or soy milk. This won't count against the other 1 cup of milk you're allowed for the day.

- Bread is allowed during this cycle. Lite is best. Use whole wheat, multigrain, seven-grain, or similar. DON'T eat white bread. When bread is allowed, you can have the equivalent of 2 thin slices or 1 whole-grain/multigrain English muffin. NO bagels.
- You can have condiments with your meals. Choose 2 items below per meal, or break them up over several meals:

  Mustard: 1 teaspoon

  Mayo: 1 teaspoon

  Ketchup: 1 teaspoon

  Relish: 1 teaspoon

  Salsa: ¼ cup

  Hot sauce: 2 tablespoons
- Limit your consumption of pineapple, watermelon, and avocado, because they have a high number on the glycemic index.
- NO white rice, white potato, or baked beans.
- The exercise program is critical to your success. You MUST do the exercise for optimal results. The daily required amounts are the *minimum* that you must do. If you want to do more, that's GREAT! Consider these extra minutes bonus dollars. The more you do, the more bonus dollars you collect!
- When you have a "two-a-day," which means two different exercise periods in a day, try to separate them by at least 6 hours for maximum effectiveness. This will help your metabolism stay elevated for a greater part of the day.
- On REST DAYS, you are not required to do any of the regimented exercises. However, stay active by walking around and keeping busy. Remember, you can still do exercise on rest days. Those calories you burn will be like collecting bonus dollars. What would it hurt to do 25 minutes of exercise even on a rest day? This brings you closer to your goal!

Day 1

MEALS

BREAKFAST

1 cup of cooked oatmeal (if you use instant or flavored, 1 packet)

1 piece of fruit (any type) **OR** 1 cup of freshly squeezed fruit or
   vegetable juice

β: *½ cup of cooked oatmeal*

γ: *½ cup of cooked oatmeal*

MEAL #2

1 fresh fruit smoothie (<200 calories)

OR

1 whey protein shake (<200 calories)

MEAL #3

1 small salad with 1 chopped hard-boiled egg

MEAL #4

1 cup of brown rice or ½ cup of cooked quinoa

2 servings of vegetables

β: *½ cup of brown rice*

γ: *½ cup of brown rice*

EXERCISE

55 minutes of cardio

Here's something you might try:

- 20 minutes of treadmill (alternate between running and
  walking: 5 walk, 2 run, 3 walk, 2 run, 5 walk, 3 run)
- 20 minutes of elliptical (10 forward, 5 reverse, 5 forward)
- 15 minutes of stationary bike (keep heart rate in fat-burning
  zone)

For those who don't have a membership to a gym:

- 30-minute walk in the neighborhood
- 10 flights of stairs
- 15 minutes of aerobics

β: 60 *minutes of cardio*

γ: 65 *minutes of cardio*

Dr. Ian's Tip

Too many people mistakenly think that because alcohol is a liquid, it won't do much to their waistline. Nothing could be further from the truth. In fact, the calories in alcoholic beverages can be sneaky and fattening at the same time. Take a look at the numbers. For 1 gram of fat, there are 9 calories. For 1 gram of carbohydrate, there are 4 calories. For 1 gram of alcohol, there are 7 calories. Did you ever think that a glass of alcohol could be almost as fattening as french fries? And there's another hidden danger with alcohol—it can lower your resistance to eat bad foods or drink more calories.

Dr. Ian's Tip

Walk and talk. If you work in an office building, try to schedule at least one meeting a day with your colleagues as a "walking meeting." If the weather is nice, go outside and enjoy the fresh air. If that's not possible, simply walk within the building and try tackling a couple of sets of stairs in the process.

Day 1 Journal Entry

BREAKFAST

Time _____

Foods _____

MEAL #2

Time _____

Foods _____

MEAL #3

Time _____

Foods _____

MEAL #4

Time _____

Foods _____

SNACKS

Time _____   Time _____   Time _____

Type and quantity _____

_____

EXERCISE

Time _____   Time _____

Types and duration _____

_____

_____

Notes _____

_____

_____

Day 2

MEALS

BREAKFAST

1–1½ cups of cold cereal with low-fat, fat free, or soy milk. (Total, Cheerios, corn flakes, Puffed Wheat, Shredded Wheat, All-Bran, and similar cereals are recommended. Stay away from presweetened cereals such as Froot Loops, Frosted Flakes, Raisin Bran, Honey Smacks, etc.)

OR

1 egg white omelet (2 egg whites or ½ cup of Egg Beaters)

1 cup of freshly squeezed juice OR 1 piece of fruit

β: *1 cup of cereal*

γ: *1 cup of cereal*

MEAL #2

6 ounces of low-fat, plain yogurt with sliced fresh fruit

MEAL #3

4 ounces of fish, chicken, turkey, or lean sirloin

1 serving of vegetables

MEAL #4

1 cup of brown rice

1 cup of beans, chickpeas, or lentils

1 serving of vegetables

β: *½ cup of brown rice; ½ cup of beans, chickpeas, or lentils*

γ: *½ cup of brown rice; ½ cup of beans, chickpeas, or lentils*

EXERCISE

35 minutes of cardio in the morning

30 minutes of cardio in the late afternoon or evening

β: 40 *minutes of cardio in the morning, 35 minutes of cardio in the afternoon or evening*

γ: 45 *minutes of cardio in the morning, 40 minutes of cardio in the afternoon or evening*

Dr. Ian's Tip

Plan ahead for a busy day. If you're going to be busy at work and you know it might be difficult consuming all of your meals at the right times, bring some healthy snacks that you can keep at your desk or in your locker. Try a small box of raisins, a small fruit cup, a couple of whole wheat crackers, a hard-boiled egg, or instant vegetable soup. Planning ahead will prevent you from giving in to the temptation of visiting the sugar-filled vending machine.

Day 2 Journal Entry

BREAKFAST

Time _____

Foods _____

MEAL #2

Time _____

Foods _____

MEAL #3

Time _____

Foods _____

MEAL #4

Time _____

Foods _____

SNACKS

Time _____   Time _____   Time _____

Type and quantity _____

_____

EXERCISE

Time _____   Time _____

Types and duration _____

_____

_____

Notes _____

_____

_____

Day 3

MEALS

BREAKFAST

1–1½ cups of cold cereal with low-fat, fat free, or soy milk. (Total, Cheerios, corn flakes, Puffed Wheat, Shredded Wheat, All-Bran, and similar cereals are recommended. Stay away from presweetened cereals such as Froot Loops, Frosted Flakes, Raisin Bran, Honey Smacks, etc.).

1 piece of any type of fruit **OR** 1 cup of freshly squeezed fruit or vegetable juice

β: *1 cup of cereal*

γ: *1 cup of cereal*

MEAL #2

1 small salad (optional: 1 chopped hard-boiled egg)

MEAL #3

1 serving of vegetables

1 cup of boiled brown rice

β: *½ cup of boiled brown rice*

γ: *½ cup of boiled brown rice*

MEAL #4

½ cup of beans, chickpeas, or lentils

1 serving of vegetables

½ cup boiled brown rice

γ: *no rice*

EXERCISE

REST DAY

β: 30 *minutes of cardio*

γ: 35 *minutes of cardio*

Dr. Ian's Tip

If you're ever feeling hungry between meals and you've already had a snack or you're trying to avoid eating a snack, grab your toothbrush and dental floss. Brush your teeth with toothpaste that has a strong peppermint flavor. You can even floss your teeth for good measure. This will dampen your urge to eat.

Day 3 Journal Entry

BREAKFAST

Time _____

Foods _____

MEAL #2

Time _____

Foods _____

MEAL #3

Time _____

Foods _____

MEAL #4

Time _____

Foods _____

SNACKS

Time _____   Time _____   Time _____

Type and quantity _____

_____

EXERCISE

Time _____   Time _____

Types and duration _____

_____

_____

Notes _____

_____

_____

Day 4

MEALS

BREAKFAST

1 egg white omelet with vegetables (2 egg whites or ½ cup of Egg Beaters or 1 whole egg)

1 piece of fruit OR 1 cup of freshly squeezed fruit or vegetable juice

MEAL #2

1 sandwich: 3 ounces of turkey, chicken, or ham on 2 slices of whole-grain or whole wheat bread (½ teaspoon of mayonnaise or 1 teaspoon of mustard allowed; you can also add lettuce and sliced tomatoes)

1 cup of freshly squeezed fruit or vegetable juice

β: *½ cup of juice*

γ: *½ cup of juice*

MEAL #3

1 large vegetable salad

½ cup of beans, chickpeas, or lentils

γ: *small salad*

MEAL #4

1 large veggie burger (no bigger than 3" across)

½ cup of brown rice

EXERCISE

30 minutes of cardio in the morning

35 minutes of cardio in the afternoon or evening

β: *35 minutes in the morning, 40 minutes in the afternoon or evening*

γ: *40 minutes in the morning, 45 minutes in the afternoon or evening*

Dr. Ian's Tip

Pack a meal. Try to bring at least one meal to work with you every day. It's all about maintaining better control of your food environment and reducing the temptation to stray from the eating plan. By planning a meal (as well as your snacks) and bringing it with you, you know what you'll be eating and won't have to search for what you need to meet the meal's eating requirement. Packing your own meal means throwing out of the window the excuse, "I had to eat the french fries because that's all I could find."

Dr. Ian's Tip

Reduce your stress. Several studies have shown that stress leads to all types of bad habits, especially when it comes to eating. If you reduce your stress, you have a better chance of being successful on an eating program and losing weight. Try meditating, doing yoga, listening to your favorite music, walking, or any other activity that helps you relax. Your heart will thank you as well.

Day 4 Journal Entry

BREAKFAST

Time _____

Foods _____

MEAL #2

Time _____

Foods _____

MEAL #3

Time _____

Foods _____

MEAL #4

Time _____

Foods _____

SNACKS

Time _____   Time _____   Time _____

Type and quantity _____

_____

EXERCISE

Time _____   Time _____

Types and duration _____

_____

_____

Notes _____

_____

_____

Day 5

MEALS

BREAKFAST

two 3" pancakes OR two 3" waffles (use no more than 1 table-spoon of oil)

1 cup of freshly squeezed juice

β:*1 pancake or 1 waffle*

γ:*1 pancake or 1 waffle*

MEAL #2

6 ounces of plain, low-fat yogurt

1 piece of fruit

MEAL #3

1 large veggie burger (3" across)

OR

1 sandwich: 3 ounces of turkey, chicken, or ham on 2 slices of bread except for white bread or white pita (1 teaspoon of mustard or ½ teaspoon of mayo, if desired; you can add lettuce and tomatoes)

MEAL #4

4 ounces of fish, chicken, turkey, or lean sirloin

2 servings of vegetables

β: *1½ servings of vegetables*

γ: *1½ servings of vegetables*

EXERCISE

60 minutes of cardio:

25 minutes on the stationary bike (keep heart rate in fat-burning zone).

25 minutes on the treadmill (incline at 3.0, speed at 3.5; when you're running, keep the incline at 3.0, or lower it to 2.0 and increase the speed to 4.0–4.5). Try running for at least 10 of the 25 minutes. They don't have to be 10 consecutive minutes, but the running segments should equal 10 minutes.

10 minutes on the elliptical.

Remember: you can decide to do as much of each activity as you prefer. If you want to do more on the bike and less on the treadmill or you don't have access to the elliptical, then make the necessary adjustments. But you MUST get 60 minutes in today.

β: *65 minutes of cardio*

γ: *70 minutes of cardio*

Dr. Ian's Tip

Eating out can be treacherous when trying to lose weight, as many of the hidden cooking ingredients are high in calories and the portion sizes tend to be way too large. Instead of eating everything on your plate, divide your food in half before you even start eating. Eat only half of what you've been served and share the rest with a friend or ask the waiter to wrap the other half so that you can take it home.

Dr. Ian's Tip

Quick snacks. It helps having the right foods available on a moment's notice. So always keep a healthy snack at your desk or in your bag so that when the urge hits, you don't go to the vending machine and load up on sugary snacks that are high in calories and low in nutritional value. Healthy snacks include baby carrots, apples, yogurt.

Day 5 Journal Entry

BREAKFAST

Time _____

Foods _____

MEAL #2

Time _____

Foods _____

MEAL #3

Time _____

Foods _____

MEAL #4

Time _____

Foods _____

SNACKS

Time _____   Time _____   Time _____

Type and quantity _____

_____

EXERCISE

Time _____   Time _____

Types and duration _____

_____

_____

Notes _____

_____

_____

Day 6

MEALS

BREAKFAST

1 cup of cooked oatmeal (if you use instant or flavored, 1 packet)

1 cup of freshly squeezed fruit or vegetable juice

β: ½ cup of cooked oatmeal

γ: ½ cup of cooked oatmeal

MEAL #2

1 small fruit smoothie (<200 calories)

OR

1 small whey protein shake (<200 calories)

MEAL #3

½ cup of cooked beans, chickpeas, or lentils

1 cup of brown rice

1 serving of vegetables

β: no brown rice

γ: no brown rice

MEAL #4

4 ounces of fish, chicken, turkey, or lean sirloin

½ large baked sweet potato

1 serving of vegetables

EXERCISE

REST DAY

β: 35 minutes of cardio

γ: 40 minutes of cardio

Dr. Ian's Tip

Low calories first. When you start eating, go for those items on your plate that are lowest in calories first. By the time you get to the higher-calorie foods, you might not be so hungry and could be less inclined to eat all of what remains.

Dr. Ian's Tip

Variety is the spice of your exercise life. Don't limit your exercises. Mix up your workout so that you don't get bored with the same routine. Also, switching your exercise routine is important because it keeps your body guessing. When your body grows accustomed to a routine, it's more likely to hold on to the fat and make it more difficult for you to lose weight, because it can do the exercise more efficiently and not require as many calories to burn.

Day 6 Journal Entry

BREAKFAST

Time _____

Foods _____

MEAL #2

Time _____

Foods _____

MEAL #3

Time _____

Foods _____

MEAL #4

Time _____

Foods _____

SNACKS

Time _____   Time _____   Time _____

Type and quantity _____

_____

EXERCISE

Time _____   Time _____

Types and duration _____

_____

_____

Notes _____

_____

_____

Day 7

MEALS

BREAKFAST

6 ounces of yogurt (low-fat or fat-free and NO fruit on bottom, but you can add fresh fruit)

1 piece of fruit **OR** 1 cup of freshly squeezed fruit or vegetable juice

MEAL #2

1 small fresh fruit smoothie (<200 calories)

OR

1 small protein shake (<200 calories)

MEAL #3

1 large salad with egg whites

½ cup of mixed sliced fruits

β: *small salad*

γ: *small salad*

MEAL #4

1 small veggie, soy, or tofu burger

1 cup of boiled brown rice or dirty rice

β: *½ cup of rice*

γ: *½ cup of rice*

EXERCISE

35 minutes of cardio in the morning

35 minutes of cardio in the afternoon or evening

β: *40 minutes in the morning, 40 minutes in the afternoon or evening*

γ: *45 minutes in the morning, 45 minutes in the afternoon or evening*

Dr. Ian's Tip

Oh boy, it's soy! One way to lower your calories and increase the nutritional value of some of your foods is to switch to soy. This low-cost protein source has been consumed in Eastern cultures for centuries. Soy contains fiber, minerals, and isoflavones, nutrients that can be beneficial in fighting chronic disease. Try a soy patty instead of a sausage patty and you'll cut the calories in half and more than double the nutritional punch. Good sources of soy include tofu, soy milk, edamame, and soybeans.

Dr. Ian's Tip

Exercise at your desk. Stack a couple of books underneath your feet while seated and put the balls of your feet on the edge of the books. Simultaneously lift up both heels as if you were standing on your toes. Do 10 toe raises, then take a minute to rest before doing another set. This will give your calf muscles a great workout. You can also work on your abdominal muscles by contracting them for 30 seconds while breathing naturally. Do this at least 15 times throughout the day.

Day 7 Journal Entry

BREAKFAST

Time _____

Foods _____

MEAL #2

Time _____

Foods _____

MEAL #3

Time _____

Foods _____

MEAL #4

Time _____

Foods _____

SNACKS

Time _____   Time _____   Time _____

Type and quantity _____

_____

EXERCISE

Time _____   Time _____

Types and duration _____

_____

_____

Notes _____

_____

_____

CHAPTER 8

Cycle 3

CONGRATULATIONS! You have made it to the final cycle of the rotation. Take a moment and give yourself credit. You have pushed yourself hard the last two weeks, and you've remained focused on your goal. This has required a lot of dedication and perseverance, and for this you deserve recognition. But the journey is not over yet. For many who will be completing only one rotation, Cycle 3 is the home stretch. Have you ever watched a long-distance race? The runners move along at incredible speeds over a long period of time, pushing their bodies and minds beyond pain and the temptation to stop and rest. But inevitably, near the end of the race when these runners look like they'll drop from exhaustion at any moment, pain etched across their faces, they dig deep and find a reserve of untapped energy that lets them kick into a sprint the last few hundred yards with the finish line in sight. Their minds take over and they are running on sheer willpower and adrenaline.

The length of time you exercise picks up in Cycle 3, but you should match that with an increase in intensity. For example, if you're currently walking on the treadmill at 3.0 mph, turn it up 10 percent to 3.3 mph. If you've been riding the stationary bike at level 7, switch to level 8. Bottom line, you're in the home stretch, which means you have to crank it up rather than turn it down. Pay specific attention to the pedometer requirement for each day. Remember, don't wear the pedometer during your specific exercise period. Wear it at all other times, such as around the house, walking in the neighborhood or mall, or any other time during the day, but not while you are fulfilling the specific cardio exercise requirement. Every step you take and every stair you climb will bring you closer to your goal.

Your body has shed a considerable amount of weight in a short period of time. It is not happy that you've changed its "fat environment," which it had grown comfortable with. Your body will now do everything in its power to work against your continued efforts to **SMASH** the fat, because its "weight set point" has been changed. Think of the weight set point as a narrow weight range where the body feels most comfortable and thus works extremely hard against your efforts to drop your weight beneath it. You can become frustrated, because even while you are eating and exercising right, your body is still holding on to the excess weight. Not to worry, this last cycle will arm you with weapons that your body can't handle and you *will* win the battle. Because this is the last of the three cycles and you're facing the most resistance you've ever faced from your body, you will need to push a little harder. You'll need to find that reserve that the long-distance runners tap into at the end of a long race. The finish line is within sight. You have only 7 days left to complete this successful rotation. Don't let anything or anyone get in the way of your breaking that tape at the finish line. Victory is within your grasp!

CYCLE 3 GUIDELINES

PLEASE READ CAREFULLY

- You're allowed up to 2 snacks each day. The snacks must be 100 calories or less. You don't have to eat snacks; it's up to you. But if you do, follow the guidelines. Remember, snacks are a great way to keep your body properly fueled throughout the day so that you can continue to reach peak performance.

- You can have 3 tablespoons of low-fat or fat-free salad dressing a day.
- You can drink up to 2 cans of diet soda per day, but remember that less is more.
- You can drink up to ½ cup of lemon juice per day.
- You can drink up to 1 cup of low-fat, fat-free, or soy milk per day, whether it's in your cereal or by itself. The milk you use in your protein shake or smoothie doesn't count against this 1 cup total.
- Drink as much plain water as you like and at any time of the day. I recommend that you drink at least 6 cups per day.
- You're allowed to have 2 SMALL cups (8 ounces) of coffee and 1 SMALL cup of tea each day.
- You're allowed to have two 6-ounce glasses of wine for the entire week. You're allowed to have three 12-ounce bottles or cans of beer and 1 mixed drink this week. Try to drink lite beer. Remember, the less alcohol you drink, the more room you'll have for other, more important calories.
- 1 vegetable serving is roughly the size of a small fist.
- Your vegetables can be steamed, grilled, boiled, or raw. You can also cook them with a little oil or butter spray.
- All protein shakes and fruit smoothies should be less than 200 calories.
- Salt is allowed, but try to keep it to no more than 1 teaspoon per day.
- Turkey and chicken are to be baked, roasted, boiled, or grilled and eaten without the skin. Avoid fried food as much as possible.

- Add some flavor to your veggies or rice by adding 1–2 tablespoons of soy sauce.
- For your fruits, load up on berries. They're full of vitamins and antioxidants. Apples, oranges, and pears are full of healthy fiber.
- If your stomach is rumbling between meals, try chewing a stick of sugarless gum. You can have unlimited carrots and celery between meals. This can help carry you until your next meal.
- 4 ounces is roughly the size of a deck of cards.
- You can have 3 tablespoons of low-fat cottage cheese per day.
- You can have 1 tablespoon of peanut butter per day.
- With your cereals, you're allowed sliced fruit/berries, ½ teaspoon of sugar, 1 teaspoon of sugar substitute. If you're eating hot cereal, you can have ½ pat of butter.
- With your protein shakes, if you're using milk instead of water, use low-fat, skim, or soy milk. This won't count against the other 1 cup of milk you're allowed for the day.
- Bread is allowed during this cycle. Lite is best. Use whole wheat, multigrain, seven-grain, or similar. DON'T eat white bread. When bread is allowed, you can have the equivalent of 2 thin slices or 1 whole-grain/multigrain English muffin. NO bagels.
- You can have condiments with your meals. Choose 2 items below per meal, or break them up over several meals:
    Mustard: 1 teaspoon
    Mayo: 1 teaspoon
    Ketchup: 1 teaspoon
    Relish: 1 teaspoon
    Salsa: ¼ cup
    Hot sauce: 2 tablespoons
- Limit your consumption of pineapple, watermelon, and avocado.
- NO white rice, white potato, or baked beans.

- The exercise program is critical to your success. You MUST do the exercise for optimal results. The daily required amounts are the *minimum* that you must do. If you want to do more, that's GREAT! Consider these extra minutes bonus dollars. The more you do, the more bonus dollars you collect!

- When you have a "two-a-day," which means two different exercise periods in a day, try to separate them by at least 6 hours for maximum effectiveness. This will help your metabolism stay elevated for a greater part of the day.

- On REST DAYS, you are not required to do any of the regimented exercises. However, stay active by walking around and keeping busy. Remember, you can still do exercise on rest days. Those calories you burn will be like collecting bonus dollars. What would it hurt to do 25 minutes of exercise even on a rest day? This brings you closer to your goal!

Day 1

MEALS

BREAKFAST

6 ounces of plain, low-fat yogurt

1 piece of fruit

MEAL #2

1 small fresh smoothie (<200 calories)

OR

1 small whey protein shake (<200 calories)

MEAL #3

½ cup of brown rice

½ cup of beans, lentils, or chickpeas

1 serving of vegetables

β: *no brown rice*

γ: *no brown rice*

MEAL #4

2 servings of vegetables

½ cup of boiled brown or dirty rice

EXERCISE

60 minutes of cardio

Pedometer: 12,000 steps

β: *70 minutes of cardio, which you can split into different sessions*

γ: *75 minutes of cardio, which you can split into different sessions*

Dr. Ian's Tip

The right soups can be your friend. Eating soups that contain chicken, beans, and/or vegetables can fill you up, provide a tasty meal, and load you up on vitamins and other healthy nutrients. As a general rule, the clearer the soup, the fewer calories it's likely to have. Avoid adding bacon bits, cheese, crackers, and cream, which all pile on unnecessary calories. Soups can be great low-calorie meals.

Dr. Ian's Tip

Weekly goals for exercise: Too often we get bogged down with long-term goals. One of the best ways to succeed on an exercise program is to set weekly goals. There are all kinds of attainable goals you can set: complete four 45-minute workouts, ride 3 miles on a bicycle during 3 different sessions, jog for half of the time you spend on the treadmill. The idea is to set smaller goals each week so that they will help you build to your larger goals. If you reach your goals for the week, treat yourself to a reward such as a massage or a new top you've been eyeing for your wardrobe.

Day 1 Journal Entry

BREAKFAST

Time _____

Foods _____

MEAL #2

Time _____

Foods _____

MEAL #3

Time _____

Foods _____

MEAL #4

Time _____

Foods _____

SNACKS

Time _____   Time _____   Time _____

Type and quantity _____

_____

EXERCISE

Time _____   Time _____

Types and duration _____

_____

_____

Notes _____

_____

_____

Day 2

MEALS

BREAKFAST

1–1½ cups of cold cereal with low-fat, fat free, or soy milk. (Total, Cheerios, corn flakes, Puffed Wheat, Shredded Wheat, All-Bran, and similar cereals are recommended. Stay away from presweetened cereals such as Froot Loops, Frosted Flakes, Raisin Bran, Honey Smacks, etc.)

1 cup of freshly squeezed vegetable or fruit juice **OR** 1 piece of fruit

β: *1 cup of cereal*

½ cup of freshly squeezed juice

γ: *1 cup of cereal*

½ cup of freshly squeezed juice

MEAL #2

1 cup of mixed fresh fruit

8 ounces or more of water

MEAL #3

½ cup of beans, chickpeas, or lentils

1 small salad

MEAL #4

1 small veggie burger **OR** 2 small soy patties (try Boca or Yves Veggie Cuisine)

½ cup of boiled brown rice **OR** 1 serving of vegetables

EXERCISE

40 minutes of cardio

Pedometer: 14,000 steps

β: *50 minutes of cardio*

γ: *60 minutes of cardio*

Dr. Ian's Tip

Improve the quality of your calories by switching from butter to olive oil. When your waiter delivers your bread basket, get rid of the mound of frozen butter and ask for some olive oil instead. This will not only add more taste to your bread, but you'll consume less of it because it's so flavorful. Olive oil is full of unsaturated (good) fats while butter is full of saturated (bad) fats. Olive oil has also been shown to be much healthier for your heart.

Dr. Ian's Tip

Most people on a diet are going to reach for a dessert every once in a while. That's fine, but make a smart decision while doing so. When dining out, if you plan on having a dessert, then skip the appetizer and the bread basket. It's all about compromise. If that sweet tooth is really aching, make the trade and leave with a smile on your face.

Day 2 Journal Entry

BREAKFAST

Time _____

Foods _____

MEAL #2

Time _____

Foods _____

MEAL #3

Time _____

Foods _____

MEAL #4

Time _____

Foods _____

SNACKS

Time _____   Time _____   Time _____

Type and quantity _____

_____

EXERCISE

Time _____   Time _____

Types and duration _____

_____

_____

Notes _____

_____

_____

Day 3

MEALS

BREAKFAST

1 cup of cooked oatmeal (if you use instant or flavored, 1 packet)

1 piece of fruit **OR** 1 cup of freshly squeezed juice

γ: *½ cup of cooked oatmeal*

MEAL #2

1 small fresh fruit smoothie (<200 calories)

OR

1 small whey protein shake (<200 calories)

MEAL #3

1 sandwich: 3 ounces of turkey, chicken, or ham on any 2 slices of bread except for white bread or white pita (1 teaspoon of mustard or ½ teaspoon of mayo, if desired; you can add lettuce and tomatoes)

1 piece of fruit

½ cup of bean soup (from a can or fresh and cooked in broth or water)

β: *no bean soup*

γ: *no bean soup*

MEAL #4

1 cup of boiled brown or dirty rice

2 servings of vegetables

1 small salad

β: *½ cup of boiled rice*

γ: *½ cup of boiled rice*

EXERCISE

40 minutes of cardio in the morning

30 minutes of cardio in the afternoon or evening

Pedometer: 12,000 steps

β: 45 *minutes in the morning, 35 minutes in the afternoon or evening*

γ: 50 *minutes in the morning, 40 minutes in the afternoon or evening*

Dr. Ian's Tip

Go shopping after you eat. Shopping while hungry will prompt you to purchase more out of immediate gratification than necessity. Also, when you're hungry, you're more inclined to give in to temptation and pick up fattening foods that are not part of your healthy eating plan.

Dr. Ian's Tip

Eat multiple small meals and help increase your metabolism. It doesn't sound right at first, but eating can actually *speed up* the metabolism that burns calories. It's called the thermogenic effect of food (TEF) and it simply means that food requires some amount of energy to be digested. It's believed that TEF represents about 5–10 percent of your total caloric expenditure for the day. Protein-rich foods tend to have a higher TEF, which means they speed up the metabolism more. So eat smaller, multiple meals and burn more calories than you would eating the traditional three larger "square" meals per day.

Day 3 Journal Entry

BREAKFAST

Time _____

Foods _____

MEAL #2

Time _____

Foods _____

MEAL #3

Time _____

Foods _____

MEAL #4

Time _____

Foods _____

SNACKS

Time _____   Time _____   Time _____

Type and quantity _____

_____

EXERCISE

Time _____   Time _____

Types and duration _____

_____

_____

Notes _____

_____

_____

Day 4

MEALS

BREAKFAST

1 egg white omelet with veggies and 1 ounce (approximately 1½
    slices) of regular or low-fat cheese (use 2 egg whites or ½ cup
    of Egg Beaters or 1 whole egg)

1 piece of fruit **OR** 1 cup of freshly squeezed juice

MEAL #2

1 small salad

1 cup of freshly squeezed fruit or vegetable juice

β: *½ cup of juice*

γ: *½ cup of juice*

MEAL #3

½ cup of boiled brown rice

2 servings of vegetables

MEAL #4

4 ounces of fish or chicken

½ cup of boiled rice

1 serving of vegetables

γ: *no rice*

EXERCISE

60 minutes of cardio

Pedometer: 14,000 steps

β: *70 minutes of cardio*

γ: *80 minutes of cardio*

Dr. Ian's Tip

The one-minute breakfast. If you're always on the go first thing in the morning, you need only a minute to get some nutrition to start your day in a positive way. Try these one-minute breakfasts: instant oatmeal topped with fruit, a bowl of yogurt and berries, a bowl of cold cereal with sliced banana or strawberries, a healthy fruit smoothie you can make in your blender.

Day 4 Journal Entry

BREAKFAST

Time _____

Foods_____

MEAL #2

Time _____

Foods_____

MEAL #3

Time _____

Foods_____

MEAL #4

Time _____

Foods_____

SNACKS

Time _____   Time _____   Time _____

Type and quantity _____

_____

EXERCISE

Time _____   Time _____

Types and duration _____

_____

_____

Notes _____

_____

_____

Day 5

MEALS

BREAKFAST

6 ounces of plain, low-fat yogurt

1 piece of fruit OR 1 cup of freshly squeezed fruit or vegetable juice

MEAL #2

1 small mixed fruit cup (all types of fruit allowed)

OR

1 small fresh fruit smoothie (<200 calories)

OR

1 small whey protein shake (<200 calories)

MEAL #3

1 sandwich: 3 ounces of turkey, chicken, or ham on any 2 slices of bread except for white bread or white pita (1 teaspoon of mustard or ½ teaspoon of mayo, if desired; you can add lettuce and tomatoes and 1 slice of cheese)

1 serving of raw or cooked vegetables

MEAL #4

½ cup of boiled brown or dirty rice

2 servings of vegetables

EXERCISE

REST DAY

Pedometer: 10,000 steps

β: 35 *minutes of cardio*

γ: 45 *minutes of cardio*

Dr. Ian's Tip

Watery foods are the way to go. Eating foods that have high water content can be a great way to lose weight. Watery foods allow you to eat as much as or even more than the calorie-rich foods and still get full on fewer calories. Foods that fit the bill include celery, cucumbers, lettuce, tomatoes, and squash.

Day 5 Journal Entry

BREAKFAST

Time _____

Foods _____

MEAL #2

Time _____

Foods _____

MEAL #3

Time _____

Foods _____

MEAL #4

Time _____

Foods _____

SNACKS

Time _____   Time _____   Time _____

Type and quantity _____

_____

EXERCISE

Time _____   Time _____

Types and duration _____

_____

_____

Notes _____

_____

_____

Day 6

MEALS

BREAKFAST

1–1½ cups of cold cereal with low-fat, fat-free, or soy milk

1 piece of fruit OR 1 cup of freshly squeezed vegetable or fruit juice

β: *1 cup of cereal*

γ: *1 cup of cereal*

MEAL #2

1 small salad

MEAL #3

½ cup of boiled brown rice

2 servings of vegetables

MEAL #4

1 veggie burger OR 4 ounces of fish, chicken, or turkey

½ cup of boiled brown rice OR 1 serving of vegetables

γ: *no rice*

EXERCISE

40 minutes in the morning

35 minutes in the afternoon or evening

Pedometer: 12,000 steps

β: *45 minutes in the morning, 40 minutes in the afternoon or evening*

γ: *50 minutes in the morning, 45 minutes in the afternoon or evening*

Dr. Ian's Tip

One way to keep cravings at bay between meals is to get a bag of ice chips and chew on them. Water has no calories, and the crunching of the ice can actually trick your body into believing it's eating something to quench the hunger pangs.

Day 6 Journal Entry

BREAKFAST

Time _____

Foods _____

MEAL #2

Time _____

Foods _____

MEAL #3

Time _____

Foods _____

MEAL #4

Time _____

Foods _____

SNACKS

Time _____   Time _____   Time _____

Type and quantity _____

_____

EXERCISE

Time _____   Time _____

Types and duration _____

_____

_____

Notes _____

_____

_____

Day 7

MEALS

BREAKFAST

1 cup of cooked oatmeal (if you use instant or flavored, 1 packet)

1 piece of fruit **OR** 1 cup of freshly squeezed vegetable or fruit juice

γ: *½ cup of cooked oatmeal*

MEAL #2

1 small fresh fruit smoothie (<200 calories)

OR

1 small whey protein shake (<200 calories)

MEAL #3

1 small salad

½ cup of beans, lentils, or chickpeas

β: *no beans*

γ: *no beans*

MEAL #4

½ cup of brown rice

3 servings of vegetables

γ: *2 servings of vegetables*

EXERCISE

35 minutes of cardio in the morning

40 minutes of cardio in the afternoon or evening

Pedometer: 15,000 steps

β: *40 minutes in the morning, 45 minutes in the afternoon or evening*

γ: *45 minutes in the morning, 50 minutes in the afternoon or evening*

Day 7 Journal Entry

BREAKFAST

Time _____

Foods _____

MEAL #2

Time _____

Foods _____

MEAL #3

Time _____

Foods _____

MEAL #4

Time _____

Foods _____

SNACKS

Time _____   Time _____   Time _____

Type and quantity _____

_____

EXERCISE

Time _____   Time _____

Types and duration _____

_____

_____

Notes _____

_____

_____

CHAPTER 9

Maintenance Phase

If you are entering MAINTENANCE, that means you have found success and you're satisfied with your results. MAINTENANCE is designed to help you keep the weight off, yet you continue to eat and exercise in a healthy way that doesn't stress you but makes you feel comfortable. The purpose of going through the cycles was not only to lose weight in a short period of time but also to learn good eating and exercise habits that will last you a lifetime. This phase is the beginning of implementing those lifestyle changes you've learned and benefited from while reaching your weight-loss goal. And now you'll have more freedom to eat out, rather than needing to prepare so many meals at home.

MAINTENANCE works because you are now able to make smart food decisions almost as second nature. For example, if you want some ice cream, you'll now opt for a low-fat version and eat only a couple of scoops rather than an entire pint at one sitting. If you have a sweet tooth and want some chocolate chip cookies, before you might've eaten an entire sleeve or bag of the cookies, but now you'll be satisfied with just a few of them. If you still have a craving even after treating yourself, reach for a piece of fruit instead of cookies. The bottom line is that you worked extremely hard to

Dr. Ian's Tip

Fresh is best! Whether it's juice or whole fruit, it's best to eat your foods as fresh as possible. Canned fruit and juices have a lot of additives and sweeteners that pack in unnecessary calories. With fresh fruit, you save on some calories and benefit from all of the natural vitamins and other nutrients the food contains.

make it to this point, so why give it all back by making poor decisions and not taking care of yourself?

I've written the MAINTENANCE phase as general guidelines that you can follow, rather than the detailed daily plans that you found in the rotation itself. I did this for a specific purpose. I don't want you to feel restricted during MAINTENANCE; rather, I prefer that *you* choose what *you* want to eat and how much *you* want to exercise and feel good about doing it. What I have provided on top of the guidelines are reminders of what you should and shouldn't do to protect your weight loss and keep you going forward instead of backward. If you don't see something on the food or drinks list, that doesn't mean you can't have it. It means that you must employ good decision making in the spirit of what you've already learned and decide on a case-by-case basis what individual food or activity will help you keep your weight in check.

If you notice that some of the pounds you have shed are creeping back on, don't stand by and do nothing. The key is to address

The milk switch. Get rid of the calorie-laden whole milk and switch to 1 percent. Let's say you drink 1 cup of milk (8 ounces) each day. By not changing anything you normally do except switching from whole milk to 1 percent milk, you could lose approximately 5 pounds in one year.

this situation early and directly before you find yourself facing another uphill battle. Choose one of the three cycles and go back in until you've lost the weight that came back. Once you're back down to where you want to be, return to MAINTENANCE. Remember, the cycles are always there to help you when you're in need. This style of healthy eating and exercise can keep you feeling great for the rest of your life! Now that you're in MAINTENANCE, you have greater flexibility with the cycles. You can do just half of a cycle, then go back to MAINTENANCE, or you can do two complete cycles, then return to MAINTENANCE. Try the cycle that was most effective for you or one that you felt most comfortable following. You will still practice the good habits of smaller meals and eating on a regular schedule to keep your energy levels up so that you can continue to operate at peak performance. Don't forget: Breakfast like a king, lunch like a prince, dinner like a pauper.

The following are some things that you should emphasize in your diet. These are your maximum quantities per day unless otherwise indicated.

MAINTENANCE

FRUITS

You can have any fruit you like, but try to minimize cantaloupe, watermelon, pineapple, and dates.

There is no real maximum. Try to have at least 3 servings per day.

VEGETABLES

A serving is the size of a medium fist.

3 servings per day

DAIRY

You can choose to eat all of the items on the list in one day or none or partial amounts.

2 cups of low-fat, skim, or soy milk

1.3 ounces of low-fat cheese (about 2 slices)

6 ounces of low-fat yogurt

EGGS

Choose only 1 item on the list.

2 egg whites

½ cup of Egg Beaters

1 whole egg (scrambled, boiled, or omelet)

MEATS

5–6 ounces, approximately the size of a deck and a half of playing cards

You can choose 1 item from this list. If you don't eat seafood, then you can choose 2 items from this list, but not at the same meal. For example, you might choose chicken for lunch and ground beef for dinner.

Chicken (without the skin)

Turkey (without the skin)

Ground beef (extra lean or ground sirloin)

Sirloin steak

Lamb

Ham

SEAFOOD

Choose 1 of the items listed. If you choose fish, have about 5 ounces (size of a deck and a half of playing cards). If you choose one of the other items as your serving of seafood, then follow the quantities as written. Choose only 1 serving to eat. If you don't eat meat, then you can choose 2 servings.

Salmon, snapper, tuna, halibut, striped bass, Chilean sea bass

Shrimp: 4 large

Mussels: 3 ounces

Oysters: 6–12

Clams: 3

Crab cakes: 2 (3" in diameter)

PASTA AND BREAD

If you decide to have pasta, eat it in place of a meat or seafood serving. You shouldn't have pasta more than 2–3 times a week.

Pasta: 1 cup, cooked (whole wheat is better)

When it comes to bread, less is more. If you must eat bread, avoid white; choose whole wheat, multigrain, seven-grain, etc.

Bread: 2 thin slices

1 pita

1 grinder roll

1 small baguette

Pizza: 3–4 slices/week

GRAINS

These items are full of fiber. Eat them often. These are maximum weekly quantities. Try to mix them up.

3 cups of brown rice

3 cups of wheat berries

2 cups of quinoa

3 cups of wild rice

3 cups of dirty rice

3 cups of basmati rice

3 cups of kasha

1½ cups of pearl barley

CEREALS

Hot (1 cup of cooked cereal)

Cold (1½ cups)

Oatmeal

Cream of wheat

Farina

Grits

You may choose either 1 hot or 1 cold per day, not both. Not all cereal brands are listed, but I have listed those cereals that tend to be more nutritious, have less sugar, and fewer calories per serving. Try to use 2%, 1%, fat-free, or soy milk.

Bran flakes

Chex

Cheerios

Corn flakes

BEVERAGES

Beverages can be very deceiving. They contain calories and, depending on the beverage, lots of them. I have listed some commonly enjoyed beverages and some guidelines on the amounts you should drink. Plain water is best, but it's all right to enjoy other drinks in the quantities listed here.

Freshly squeezed fruit/vegetable juice (1–2 cups per day)

Diet soda (limit of two 8-ounce cans per day)

Regular soda (limit of one 8-ounce can per day)

Coffee (1 cup–8 ounces–per day)

Water (unlimited)

Vitamin water (limit of 16 ounces per day)

Iced tea (1 cup–8 ounces–per day if sweetened; 2 cups if unsweetened)

Tea (2 cups, decaf or caffeinated)

Lemonade (1 cup–8 ounces–per day)

ALCOHOL

These are maximum amounts for a week. Many alcoholic drinks have lots of calories and also lead to eating unhealthy foods, so limit your consumption as much as possible.

Beer: three 12-ounce bottles

Wine: three 6-ounce glasses

Mixed drinks: two 6-ounce glasses

CONDIMENTS AND OTHERS

These are commonly used items. You can choose 4 of these items to eat over the course of the entire day, but try to stick to the daily maximum quantities shown.

Mustard: 1 teaspoon

Mayo: 1 teaspoon

Ketchup: 1 teaspoon

Relish: 1 teaspoon

Salsa: ¼ cup

Hot sauce: 2 tablespoons

Soy sauce: 2 tablespoons

Peanut butter: 2 tablespoons

Cottage cheese: 3 tablespoons

Jelly: 1 tablespoon

Cream cheese: 1 tablespoon

SNACKS/DESSERTS

See the snacks section that follows.

The following list contains items that are either not very healthy or are full of "wasted" calories. Just because they're on this list it doesn't mean you have to completely eliminate them; rather, reduce your consumption as much as you can. A little serving won't hurt, but more than that and you could find yourself sliding down that slippery slope of weight gain.

SMASH LIST

Cut back on these foods:

- Alcohol
- Bacon (try soy or turkey products)
- Bagels
- Brownies
- Buttered popcorn
- Cake
- Candy
- Dried fruit (tends to be high in calories; fresh is much better)
- Frappuccino or cappuccino
- French fries
- Fried foods in general (instead grill, sauté, bake, roast, steam, or boil)
- Fruit juice blends/drinks (aim for 100 percent fruit juices)
- Ice cream
- Latte
- Milk shakes
- Pastries/Danish/doughnuts
- Pizza
- Potato chips/corn chips/tortilla chips (choose low-fat versions)
- Regular soda
- Sausage (try soy or turkey products)
- White bread/English muffins
- White flour
- White pasta
- White potatoes
- White rice
- Whole milk

EXERCISE

Just because you're in MAINTENANCE doesn't mean you give up on the exercise. For the rest of your life you should participate in some regular exercise program. This will be critical as you begin to consume more calories in MAINTENANCE. The math is very simple. If you're adding calories to your diet, you must figure out how to burn them off so that these excess calories don't get stored as fat.

Cardio exercises are the best at fat burning, but you should also develop a regular program of either light free-weight lifting or resistance exercises to increase your lean muscle mass. I recommend during this phase that at the minimum you do 3 days of cardio for at least 45 minutes each session. Twice during the week you should work on building your lean muscle mass. You can work on your muscles on the same days you do your cardio, or on separate days. It doesn't make a difference. The key, however, is to do both to maximize your fat-burning capacity and boost your metabolism. If you want to have a more intense exercise program even during MAINTENANCE, then all the better.

Here's what a sample week might look like. You can do more if you like, but at the minimum, try something like this.

Monday	45 minutes of cardio
Tuesday	45 minutes of free weights/ resistance bands
Wednesday	Rest
Thursday	45 minutes of cardio
Friday	30 minutes of free weights/ resistance bands
Saturday	Rest
Sunday	45 minutes of cardio

You have worked EXTREMELY hard to reach your goals and get yourself to a place where you can do a better job of maintaining a healthy weight and lifestyle. You have demonstrated that you have the desire and willpower to succeed. Now it's time to enjoy the hard-earned fruits of your labor and not give them back!

CHAPTER 10

Snacks

Snacks can be extremely helpful on this or any other program if used correctly. The concept of snacking boils down to consuming a smaller amount of food in between larger meals to quench those hunger pangs that can creep up as your body is waiting for its next hit of calories. A snack is *not* a meal, and you shouldn't think about it that way. Snacks can become a detriment rather than a benefit when you start consuming them for reasons other than what's intended or beyond the allowable quantities. Just because these foods typically come in smaller portions, it doesn't mean they are calorie-free. Snacks contain calories, and the more you eat of even the lowest-calorie snack, the greater the number of calories you're putting into your body. Remember, a snack is just meant to carry you over until that next meal, not to be a meal in and of itself.

This section contains a list of snacks that are roughly 100 calories each. You can choose any snack, but limit yourself to 2 snacks each day. In fact, if you're eating all of the meals as laid out in the plan, you won't want to eat more than 2 snacks per day, because you won't be hungry.

- ½ protein bar (like Balance or Power Bar)
- half an apple with 2 teaspoons of peanut butter

- orange and a few dry-roasted nuts
- 10 cashews
- 12 almonds
- ½ small avocado
- 4 mini rice cakes with 2 tablespoons of low-fat cottage cheese
- 3 ounces of low-fat cottage cheese and 3 whole wheat crackers
- 3 tablespoons of fat-free salad dressing with mixed raw veggies
- 10 chocolate-covered raisins
- 6 Wheat Thins crackers with 2 teaspoons of peanut butter
- ½ cup of applesauce and 1 piece of whole wheat toast cut into four sticks for dunking
- ½ cup of frozen orange juice or grape juice, eaten as sorbet
- 2 crumbled vanilla wafers and 1 scoop of low-fat whipped topping
- 2 large graham cracker squares with 1 teaspoon of peanut butter
- 8 animal crackers
- 2 cups of unbuttered, air-popped popcorn
- ½ cup of sugar-free gelatin, any flavor, and 1 tablespoon of low-fat whipped topping
- 4–6 ounces of fat-free or low-fat yogurt (unsweetened)
- ½ cup of fat-free ice cream
- 1 ounce of string cheese with 4 whole wheat crackers
- 6 ounces of tossed salad with lettuce, tomato, and cucumber, and 3 tablespoons of fat-free dressing
- 5 saltine crackers or 2 graham cracker squares with 2 tablespoons of peanut butter
- Place a marshmallow on top of a graham cracker and heat in the microwave until soft, pour on 1 teaspoon of chocolate syrup
- 25 grapes
- 8-ounce fat-free chocolate pudding cup
- 1 hard-boiled egg sprinkled with a dash of salt and pepper
- one 2" slice of angel food cake

- 2 tablespoons of roasted sunflower seeds
- 5 Hershey's Kisses
- 1 cup of blueberries
- ½ cup of unsweetened applesauce
- 1 celery stalk with 2 tablespoons of peanut butter
- ½ cup of sliced cucumbers with 3 tablespoons of fat-free dressing
- ½ cup of fruit salad
- 3 small gingersnaps
- ½ grapefruit with a sprinkle of sugar
- 1 cup of cubed honeydew melon
- 1 cup of vegetable soup with beef, chicken, or turkey
- 2 chocolate chip cookies, 2" diameter
- 5 vanilla wafers
- 12 grape tomatoes with 2 tablespoons of hummus
- 3 pieces of hard candy
- ½ cup of low-fat or fat-free sherbet
- 1 cup of fresh strawberries
- 6 bite-size pieces of red or black licorice
- 1 cup of chicken noodle soup
- 6 roasted chestnuts (approximately 1 ounce out of shell)
- ½ cup of nonfat frozen yogurt
- 1 frozen fruit and juice bar
- ½ cup of water-packed fruit cocktail (drain the liquid if it's syrup)
- 9 large jelly beans
- 8 small green or black olives
- ¼ cup of cranberry sauce
- ½ cup of sliced cooked plantains
- 1 cup of mixed fresh veggies drizzled with 3 tablespoons of low-fat or fat-free dressing
- 2 Quaker rice cakes
- 2 Jell-O sugar-free gelatin snacks

- 1 Jell-O fat-free or sugar-free pudding snack
- one 3-ounce can of water-packed tuna
- ½ cup edamame (fresh soybeans), shelled
- 1 small 5.5 ounce can V8 juice
- ¼ cup wasabi peas

FREE SNACKS

- Dill pickles
- Mini carrots
- Celery sticks
- Radishes
- Jicama slices
- Pickled peppers
- Hard-boiled egg whites

CHAPTER 11

Easy and Tasty Recipes

· CHEF'S SALAD ·

SERVINGS: 1

1 hard-boiled egg
3 ounces chicken or ham
3 ounces deli-style roasted turkey
    breast
½ cup peeled, sliced cucumbers
1 cup chopped romaine lettuce

3 tomato wedges
1 carrot, peeled and grated
2 scallions, sliced
3 tablespoons reduced-fat or fat-
    free salad dressing

Cut egg into eighths.

Slice meat into narrow strips.

Combine all ingredients except dressing in a bowl and toss.

Drizzle with the salad dressing.

· CHICKEN CAESAR SALAD ·

SERVINGS: 1

3 ounces grilled or baked boneless, skinless chicken breast

1 medium green apple (Granny Smith)

2 cups chopped romaine lettuce

1 ½ tablespoons grated Parmesan cheese

3 tablespoons low-fat or fat-free salad dressing

Slice the chicken into small strips.

Cut the apple into small wedges and then toss it with the lettuce.

Add the chicken strips.

Sprinkle the salad with the Parmesan cheese and drizzle with the dressing.

· CRAB SALAD ·

SERVINGS: 1

1 tablespoon fat-free sour cream

2 teaspoons lemon juice

½ tablespoon chopped scallion

1 tablespoon light mayonnaise

2 tablespoons chopped red bell pepper

1 tablespoon 1% milk

4 ounces crabmeat (canned, frozen and thawed, or fresh)

2 cups chopped romaine lettuce

1 tablespoon minced chives

Combine the sour cream, lemon juice, scallion, mayonnaise, red pepper, and milk in a bowl and whisk.

Add the crabmeat to the dressing and mix.

Set crab mixture on top of the lettuce and sprinkle with the chives.

• GREEK CHICKEN SALAD •

SERVINGS: 1

3 ounces grilled boneless, skinless chicken breast

1 cup baby spinach leaves

½ cup chopped romaine lettuce

1 small cucumber, peeled and sliced

1 tablespoon country Dijon mustard

¾ tablespoon balsamic vinegar

1½ tablespoons grated Parmesan cheese

Cut the chicken breast into chunks.

Combine the spinach, lettuce, cucumber, and chicken in a bowl.

Add the mustard and vinegar to a small saucepan, then whisk together until smooth over low heat. Add 1 tablespoon water and whisk again. Add the Parmesan cheese to the mixture and heat until the mixture is warm.

Pour the dressing over the greens.

• EASY TOSSED SALAD •

SERVINGS: 1

¾ cup chopped romaine lettuce

¼ cup chopped tomato

¼ cup peeled and sliced cucumber

¼ cup grated carrots

2 red onion slices

3 tablespoons fat-free or low-fat salad dressing

Combine all ingredients except the salad dressing. Chill salad before serving.

Drizzle with the salad dressing.

· THREE-BEAN SALAD ·

SERVINGS: 2

¼ cup cooked dark red kidney
   beans (canned is fine)
½ cup cut green beans (fresh or
   canned)
2 red bell peppers, sliced
1 tablespoon sugar
1 tablespoon extra virgin olive oil
1 tablespoon cider vinegar

½ teaspoon minced fresh parsley
2 tablespoons ground dry
   mustard, such as Coleman's
2 tablespoons oregano
2 slices onion
1 pinch salt
½ cup fat-free or low-fat salad
   dressing

Rinse and drain canned beans and, if using, rinse fresh green beans.
Combine all ingredients in a large bowl, and toss well. Chill for 20
   minutes before serving.

· SALMON SALAD ·

SERVINGS: 1

One 5-ounce salmon fillet
¼ cup peeled and chopped
   cucumber
¼ teaspoon seasoned salt, such
   as Lawry's

3 teaspoons light mayonnaise
¼ tablespoon lemon juice
1 tablespoon low-fat sour cream
1 pinch freshly ground black
   pepper

Bake, grill, or broil the salmon until it flakes easily with a fork.
Combine the cucumber, seasoned salt, mayonnaise, lemon juice,
   sour cream, and pepper in a bowl and mix together
Dice the salmon (or cut into strips) and add to the mixture.
Serve hot or cold.

SERVINGS: 4

2 tablespoons olive oil
1 small red onion, finely chopped
2 cloves garlic, minced
2 cups brown rice, uncooked
½ teaspoon ground cumin
1 teaspoon salt
2 cups cooked black beans
    (canned, rinsed, and drained
    is fine)

1 red bell pepper, seeded and
    chopped
2 tomatoes, diced
⅓ cup chopped parsley
1 scallion, chopped
2 teaspoons balsamic vinegar
¼ teaspoon freshly ground black
    pepper

In a large saucepan with a tight-fitting lid, heat the oil over low heat.
    Add the onion and garlic and cook, with frequent stirring, for 3 to
    5 minutes.

Stir in the rice, cumin, and salt. Add 3 cups of water and bring to a
    simmer.

Turn heat down to low, cover, and cook until rice is done (15 to 20
    minutes). Uncover the rice and let it come to room temperature.

Combine the rice, beans, pepper, tomatoes, parsley, scallion, bal-
    samic vinegar, and black pepper in a bowl and toss.

SERVINGS: 4

One 15-ounce can chickpeas
(garbanzo beans), drained
1 cucumber, peeled and chopped
1 cup sliced tomatoes
¼ cup chopped onion
1 tablespoon minced garlic

½ teaspoon dried parsley flakes
¼ teaspoon dried basil
1 tablespoon grated Parmesan
cheese
1 tablespoon olive oil
3 tablespoons balsamic vinegar

In a large bowl, toss together the chickpeas, cucumber, tomatoes,
onion, garlic, parsley flakes, dried basil, and cheese.

Drizzle with the olive oil and balsamic vinegar.

Cover and refrigerate at least 30 minutes before serving.

SERVINGS: 4

Two 12-ounce cans tuna (in
water), drained
Two 15-ounce cans dark red
kidney beans (rinsed)
4 stalks celery, sliced (against
grain) ⅛ inch thick
1 red bell pepper, seeded and
roughly chopped

1 green pepper, seeded and
roughly chopped
1 medium onion (preferably
Vidalia), roughly chopped
¼ cup olive oil
¼ cup white vinegar
Freshly ground black pepper to
taste

Mix all ingredients together in a bowl.

Let sit for 10 minutes, then serve.

· CHICKEN PESTO SALAD ·

SERVINGS: 4

2 pounds boneless, skinless
chicken breast
1 teaspoon extra virgin olive oil
3 cups fresh spinach and leafy
romaine lettuce mix

FOR THE PESTO:

1 package fresh basil
1 small bunch Italian parsley
(leaves only)

¾ cup pine nuts
2 cloves garlic, minced
¼ cup grated Parmesan cheese
½ cup extra virgin olive oil
Salt and freshly ground black
pepper to taste

Trim all visible fat from chicken, and sauté breasts in 1 tablespoon
olive oil, turning to brown both sides. Sauté until cooked through
and no longer pink, about 20 minutes. Let cool.

Make the pesto: While chicken is cooking, combine the pesto ingredients in a food processor or blender. Process until smooth.

Cut the chicken into chunks, combine it with the pesto, and spoon
over plates of the spinach and lettuce mix.

• VIGOROUS BLACK BEAN SOUP •

SERVINGS: 4

Two 15-ounce cans black beans
  (undrained)
1 medium red onion, chopped
1 clove garlic, minced
½ teaspoon ground cumin

2 medium tomatoes, diced
1 tablespoon fresh cilantro,
  minced
Salt and freshly ground black
  pepper to taste

Combine the beans, onion, garlic, cumin, and tomatoes in a large
  saucepan. Cook 20 minutes over medium heat, or until onion is
  tender. Stir occasionally.

Remove from heat. If soup is too thick, add water until soup is desired consistency.

Sprinkle with cilantro, salt, and pepper just before serving.

· CURRIED SQUASH SOUP ·

SERVINGS: 5

1 small butternut squash
1 acorn squash
3 tablespoons olive oil
2 teaspoons curry powder
1 teaspoon cinnamon
1 medium onion, chopped
3 garlic cloves, minced

1 tablespoon minced fresh ginger root
5 cups chicken broth
2 tablespoons lemon juice
Salt and freshly ground black pepper to taste

Preheat the oven to 375°F.

Cut the squash in half and lay them cut side down on a lightly oiled baking sheet. Roast until the flesh is soft, 35 to 45 minutes. When the squash has cooled, scoop out the seeds and throw them away. Take a spoon and scoop out the squash flesh into a bowl.

Heat the oil in a small pan and stir in the curry powder and cinnamon. Add the chopped onion, garlic, and ginger root and sauté for 5 minutes.

Puree the squash flesh with the chicken broth and onion mixture in batches in a blender, food processor, or with a hand-held immersion blender. Add the lemon juice.

Pour the mixture into a pot and reheat it. Check the seasoning and add salt and pepper to taste.

· JULIANNA'S POTATO-LEEK SOUP ·

SERVINGS: 4

2 baking potatoes, peeled and
    roughly chopped
2 leeks (tender portions only), well
    washed, halved lengthwise,
    and chopped
1 clove garlic, peeled
32 ounces low-fat chicken broth

1 fennel bulb, chopped
4 tablespoons minced fresh
    tarragon, or 1 tablespoon
    dried
Salt and freshly ground black
    pepper to taste

Combine the potatoes, leeks, garlic, broth, and fennel in a soup pot
    and bring to a boil.

Reduce the heat and cook for 20 minutes, or until the potatoes are
    soft. Add the tarragon.

Puree the soup in batches in a blender, food processor, or with a
    hand-held immersion blender. Return the soup to the pot, reheat,
    and add salt and pepper to taste.

· GENTLE CURRIED LENTIL SOUP ·

SERVINGS: 2

1½ cups lentils
1 tablespoon olive oil
3 cups low-fat chicken broth
    (or water)
1 clove garlic, minced

1 teaspoon curry powder
1 large onion, finely chopped
1 tablespoon finely chopped
    celery

Combine all ingredients in a medium-size pot, bring to a boil, and
    cook over low heat for 30 minutes, or until lentils soften.

Serve hot.

• PARISIAN OMELET •

SERVINGS: 1

FOR THE FILLING

¼ cup peeled and diced carrot

½ tsp grated or minced fresh
  ginger root

½ teaspoon extra virgin olive oil

¼ cup zucchini, cut in 1-inch
  strips

¼ cup sliced mushrooms

1 tablespoon Worcestershire
  sauce

½ teaspoon cornstarch

FOR THE OMELET

½ teaspoon extra virgin olive oil

4 egg whites, whipped, or ⅔ cup
  Egg Beaters

1 teaspoon salt

½ teaspoon freshly ground black
  pepper

Make the vegetable filling: Cook the carrot and ginger root in olive oil for 3 minutes. Add the zucchini and mushrooms. Stir-fry until the vegetables are tender. In a mixing bowl, combine the Worcestershire sauce and cornstarch. Pour over the vegetable mixture. Toss gently to mix. Cover and keep warm.

Make the omelet: Heat the oil over medium-high heat in a skillet with a rounded bottom and sloping sides.

In a mixing bowl, whip the egg whites, 1 tablespoon water, salt, and black pepper together, using a whisk or a fork. Pour the egg mixture into the skillet. Cook over medium heat until the bottom is set. Shake the pan to loosen omelet and continue to cook 2 to 3 minutes.

Spoon the filling onto one half of the omelet. Using a spatula, fold the omelet in half over the filling. Slide the omelet out onto a plate.

SERVINGS: 2

1 teaspoon olive oil
¾ cup chopped onion
½ cup red bell pepper, seeded
  and chopped
1 clove garlic, minced
¼ cup green olives
¼ teaspoon dried oregano
½ cup shredded mozzarella
  cheese (full-fat or low-fat)

8 egg whites or 1 cup Egg
  Beaters
½ teaspoon salt
¼ teaspoon freshly ground black
  pepper

Heat a pan over medium heat. Add ½ teaspoon olive oil, the onion, bell pepper, and garlic; sauté until soft.

Add the olives and oregano; cook 1 minute or until thoroughly heated. Remove from heat; stir in cheese. Set aside.

Combine the eggs, salt, and pepper in a bowl. Stir well.

Heat ¼ teaspoon olive oil in a small nonstick pan over medium-high heat. Add half of the egg mixture to the skillet. Once the bottom is set, carefully lift the edges of the omelet with a spatula; allow uncooked portion to flow underneath cooked portion. Cook 3 minutes.

Spoon half the vegetable mixture onto the omelet. Carefully loosen with a spatula; fold omelet in half. Cook an additional minute. Slide onto a plate.

Repeat for the second omelet.

• SPINACH OMELET •

SERVINGS: 1

3 teaspoons olive oil
1 clove garlic, minced
1 small onion, minced
Half of a 10-ounce package
   chopped frozen spinach,
   thawed and drained
4 egg whites or ⅔ cup Egg
   Beaters

¼ cup 1% milk
1 pinch salt
Freshly ground black pepper to
   taste
¼ cup marinara sauce, heated

Heat the olive oil in a nonstick skillet over medium heat. Add the
   garlic and onion, and cook for 1 minute.
Add the spinach and heat through for 1 minute.
Beat the eggs with the milk, salt, and pepper and add to garlic-onion
   mixture.
Cover and cook until well set (approximately 3 minutes).
Spoon the marinara sauce over the top and serve.

• VEGETABLE AND CHEESE OMELET •

SERVINGS: 1

3 egg whites or ½ cup Egg
  Beaters
⅓ cup 1% milk
2 tablespoons chopped red bell
  pepper

¼ cup broccoli florets
1 tablespoon chopped scallion
2 ounces cheddar cheese (full-fat
  or low-fat), shredded

Combine the egg whites and milk and beat well with a whisk or a
  fork.
Pour the egg mixture into a nonstick pan.
Add the chopped vegetables and cheese to egg mixture. Cook over
  medium heat until eggs begin to bubble and the bottom is set.
Fold half of egg mixture to cover over the cheese and vegetables and
  cook another 2 to 3 minutes.

• CITRUS ZINGER FRUIT SALAD •

SERVINGS: 2

½ cup orange slices
½ cup grapes
¼ cup fresh pink grapefruit slices

¼ cup diced cantaloupe
¼ cup fresh strawberries, sliced
¼ cup fresh blueberries

Combine all ingredients in a large bowl and chill before serving.

SERVINGS: 2

2 tablespoons orange juice

½ tablespoon sugar

1 teaspoon lemon juice

½ teaspoon brown sugar

⅛ teaspoon vanilla extract

¼ cup strawberries, sliced

¼ cup peaches, peeled, pitted, and sliced

½ cup honeydew melon, peeled and diced

¼ cup blueberries

In a saucepan, combine the orange juice, sugar, 2 teaspoons water, lemon juice, and brown sugar. Mix well. Bring to a boil. Once boiling, reduce heat and simmer for 3 to 4 minutes. Remove from heat and stir in vanilla. Let cool.

In a large mixing bowl, combine the strawberries, peaches, melon, and blueberries.

Pour the cooled orange juice mixture over the fruit and toss until fruit is covered.

Cover and refrigerate for at least 6 hours. Serve cold.

• WHOLESOME WHOLE WHEAT PANCAKES •

SERVINGS: 2

1 cup flour

1 cup whole wheat flour

1 teaspoon baking powder

½ teaspoon salt

2 eggs or ½ cup Egg Beaters

2 tablespoons honey

1½ cups 1% or skim milk

¼ cup blueberries

Combine the flours, baking powder, and salt in a bowl.

Whisk the eggs, honey, and milk in a bowl.

Add the liquid to the dry ingredients. Stir until blended.

Cook on a preheated lightly greased griddle until golden brown, turning pancakes when bubbles appear in the middle of the uncooked sides.

Sprinkle blueberries on top and serve.

• PROTEINACEOUS OATMEAL •

SERVINGS: 1

1 packet Quaker Oats Apple
   Cinnamon Instant Oatmeal

1 large egg white

¼ cup 1% milk

Add water to the oatmeal, in quantity as the package recommends.

Beat the egg white with a fork and add it to the oatmeal. Mix well.

Microwave on high for 2 minutes.

Add milk to serve.

• CHICKEN CHEESE SANDWICH •

SERVINGS: 1

1 slice American cheese (full-fat
  or low-fat)
3 ounces grilled boneless,
  skinless chicken breast
1 small whole wheat hoagie roll

1 tablespoon light mayonnaise
1 romaine lettuce leaf
2 slices tomato
2 tablespoons fat-free or low-fat
  salad dressing

Melt the cheese onto the chicken breast in a microwave or oven.

Slice the hoagie roll in half and spread the mayonnaise on both halves.

Assemble the sandwich by stacking the chicken breast, lettuce, and tomato on the roll.

Drizzle the salad dressing on the tomato before closing the sandwich.

• HEALTHY ROAST BEEF SANDWICH •

SERVINGS: 1

1 tablespoon light mayonnaise

2 slices whole wheat bread

½ cup chopped spinach

2 tomato slices

3 ounces thinly sliced deli-style
  roast beef

1 slice cheese (low-fat or full-fat,
  optional)

Spread the mayo on one slice of the bread, then cover it with the
  spinach and the tomato slices.

Add the meat and close the sandwich.

Optional: Add the slice of cheese.

• HOT ROASTED THANKSGIVING SANDWICH •

SERVINGS: 1

2 slices multigrain bread

1 tablespoon light mayonnaise

1 tablespoon cranberry sauce

3 ounces sliced oven-roasted
  turkey breast

1 slice provolone cheese

2 slices tomato

Butter spray for toasting sandwich

Toast the bread, then spread the mayonnaise on one side of each
  piece of bread.

Spread cranberry sauce on one piece of bread.

Place the turkey, cheese, and tomato slices on the bread.

Cover with the remaining slice of bread.

Spray a nonstick skillet with the butter spray and toast each side of
  the sandwich over medium-high heat for no more than 2 minutes.

• BBQ TURKEY SANDWICH •

SERVINGS: 1

4 ounces sliced oven-roasted turkey breast	1 whole wheat kaiser roll, sliced in half
2 ounces barbecue sauce	1 tablespoon sweet pickle relish

Heat the turkey breast and barbecue sauce in a small saucepan over medium heat until the turkey is warmed through, approximately 3 minutes.

Place the turkey on the roll. Top with the relish and serve.

• GRILLED TURKEY REUBEN SANDWICH •

SERVINGS: 1

¼ cup shredded cabbage	3 ounces sliced oven-roasted turkey breast
1 teaspoon fat-free Thousand Island salad dressing	1 slice Swiss cheese (low-fat or full-fat)
2 teaspoons light mayonnaise	Cooking spray for toasting sandwich
½ teaspoon Dijon mustard	
2 slices rye bread	

Mix the cabbage, dressing, and mayonnaise in a small bowl.

Spread the mustard on one slice of bread. Add the turkey and the cheese. Add the cabbage mixture. Top with the remaining slice of bread.

Spray a nonstick skillet with cooking spray and toast the sandwich, flipping once, until the bread is golden brown and the cheese is melted.

• CHICKEN SALAD SANDWICH •

SERVINGS: 1

4 ounces boneless, skinless
   roasted chicken breast
2 tablespoons light mayonnaise
2 tablespoons diced celery

Salt to taste
¼ cup alfalfa sprouts (optional)
2 slices tomato
2 slices 7-grain bread

Combine the chicken, mayonnaise, diced celery, and salt in a small
   bowl to make the salad.

Assemble the sandwich, using the chicken salad, sprouts (optional),
   tomato, and bread.

• EGG SALAD SANDWICH •

SERVINGS: 1

½ cup chopped hard-boiled egg
   (about two medium-size eggs)
2 tablespoons light mayonnaise
1 pinch salt
1 pinch freshly ground black
   pepper

½ cup chopped romaine lettuce
2 slices tomato
1 whole wheat kaiser roll, sliced in
   half

Combine the chopped egg, mayonnaise, salt, and pepper to make
   the salad.

Assemble the sandwich, using the egg salad, lettuce, tomato, and
   kaiser roll.

• VEGETARIAN TURKEY SANDWICH •

SERVINGS: 1

2 slices whole wheat or 7-grain
  bread
1 tablespoon light mayonnaise
3 ounces Yves Veggie Cuisine
  Veggie Turkey Slices

1 lettuce leaf
2 slices tomato
3 slices pickled jalapeño pepper,
  or more to taste

Toast the bread and spread mayonnaise on one slice.

Assemble the sandwich, using the veggie turkey, lettuce, tomato,
  peppers, and bread.

• GRILLED SWEET PEPPER •
AND HUMMUS SANDWICH

SERVINGS: 1

2 slices whole wheat or multigrain
  bread
½ red bell pepper, seeded and
  sliced thickly
¼ yellow bell pepper, seeded and
  sliced thickly

1 thick slice onion
½ tablespoon capers
2 tablespoons hummus

Preheat a grill.

Toast the bread on the grill or in a toaster.

Grill the pepper and onion for 5 minutes, turning occasionally.

Place the vegetables and capers in a bowl and toss.

Spread the hummus on both slices of the toasted bread and assemble the sandwich, using the hot grilled vegetables.

· VEGETARIAN CLUB SANDWICH ·

SERVINGS: 1

3 slices whole wheat or 7-grain
   bread
1 tablespoon light mayonnaise
2 slices Yves Veggie Cuisine
   Sliced Canadian Bacon
1 slice Yves Veggie Cuisine
   Veggie Ham

2 slices Yves Veggie Cuisine
   Veggie Turkey
2 slices tomato
¼ cup chopped iceberg lettuce

Toast the bread and spread about 1 teaspoon mayonnaise on one
   side of each slice.
Cook the Canadian bacon in a nonstick skillet, until lightly
   browned, and slice it into strips.
Assemble all other ingredients on the toasted bread.

· LOBSTER SANDWICH ·

SERVINGS: 1

4 ounces steamed lobster, cut
   into chunks (pre-cooked
   lobster is available at many fish
   departments of grocery stores)

1 tablespoon light mayonnaise
2 slices 7-grain bread
2 slices tomato
¼ cup alfalfa sprouts

Combine the lobster with the mayonnaise.
Place the lobster mixture on one slice of the bread.
Top with the tomato slices, alfalfa sprouts, and bread.

• TASTY HALIBUT SANDWICH •

SERVINGS: 1

2 teaspoons soy sauce

2 tablespoons white wine

½ teaspoon minced or grated
   fresh ginger root

One 4-ounce halibut fillet

1 tablespoon olive oil

2 large slices onion

1 teaspoon honey

1 tablespoon light mayonnaise

1 Pepperidge Farm 7-Grain
   French Roll, sliced in half

1 romaine lettuce leaf

Preheat a broiler or a grill.

Combine one teaspoon of the soy sauce, wine, and ¼ teaspoon of the ginger root in a small bowl. Whisk together to make a marinade.

Set aside 2 tablespoons of the marinade and pour remaining marinade over the fish. Marinate for at least 20 minutes in the refrigerator.

Pour the olive oil into a nonstick skillet and add the onion. Sauté for 5 minutes over medium heat. Add the honey and the remaining teaspoon of soy sauce. Mix and keep warm.

Remove the fish from the marinade and discard excess marinade. Broil or grill for 4 to 5 minutes per side, basting with the reserved wine/soy sauce mixture.

Combine the mayonnaise and remaining ¼ teaspoon ginger root. Spread on the roll.

Assemble the sandwich, using the fish fillet, onion, lettuce, and roll. Serve hot.

• MUSHROOM ROAST •

SERVINGS: 6

One 4-pound boneless beef roast (bottom round, top round, or rump)
1 tablespoon olive oil
Three 11-ounce cans mushroom soup

6 ounces low-fat sour cream
1 cup 1% milk
1 tablespoon salt
1 tablespoon freshly ground black pepper
1 large onion, sliced

Preheat the oven to 375°F.

Divide the roast into large chunks about ½ inch thick.

Sauté the meat in a pan with olive oil, turning until all sides are brown.

Heat the soup in a separate pan and mix with the sour cream, milk, salt, and pepper.

Put the meat in a baking pan and cover with the sliced onion. Cover the meat with the soup mixture.

Bake for approximately 3 hours.

HONEY-SWEET MARINATED · GRILLED PORK CHOPS

SERVINGS: 2

FOR THE MARINADE
2 tablespoons honey
2 tablespoons orange juice
1 teaspoon brown sugar
3 tablespoons soy sauce

Two 5-ounce pork chops

Make the Marinade: Pour ½ cup water into a saucepan and bring to a simmer. Add the honey, orange juice, brown sugar, and soy sauce. Mix well and cook on low heat for 5 minutes, until reduced slightly. Let cool to room temperature.

Place the pork chops in the marinade and let sit for 2 to 3 hours, refrigerated.

Prepare a grill, preheat a broiler, or preheat the oven to 350°F.

Remove the pork chops from the marinade, then grill, broil, or bake until cooked to your preference. Use the remaining marinade to baste meat while cooking.

· GRILLED LAMB CHOPS ·

SERVINGS: 1

1 clove garlic, minced
1 heaping teaspoon country Dijon
   mustard
Salt and freshly ground black
   pepper to taste

3 rib lamb chops (or one loin lamb
   chop), trimmed of all excess fat

Preheat the broiler.

Combine the garlic, mustard, salt, and pepper and press the mixture into one side of each chop.

Broil the chops approximately 4 minutes on the coated side of the chop first and 3 minutes on the uncoated side afterward, to cook until medium doneness.

· PURE AND FLAVORFUL HAMBURGER ·

SERVINGS: 2

¾ pound ground chuck (90% lean)
1 tablespoon country Dijon mustard
1 tablespoon ketchup
1 teaspoon light mayonnaise

Salt and freshly ground black pepper to taste
2 slices tomato
2 thick slices red onion
8 slices dill pickle

Heat a grill, grill pan, or sauté pan until hot but not smoking (approximately 3 minutes).

Form the ground chuck into two loosely packed patties.

Sear the patties on both sides until browned. Then lower the heat and cook 3 minutes more on each side for medium doneness.

Combine the mustard, ketchup, mayonnaise, salt, and pepper to make a sauce.

Slather the sauce on the patties and serve topped with tomato, onion, and pickle.

· FIESTA STEAK ·

SERVINGS: 2

1 pound flank steak

3 cloves garlic, minced

2 tablespoons olive oil

Salt and freshly ground black
pepper to taste

Tomato Salsa (see page 196)

Marinate the flank steak in the garlic, olive oil, salt, and pepper for at least 30 minutes and up to overnight.

Heat a grill pan or sauté pan and sear the steak about 3 minutes each side, or until browned. Then lower heat, cover pan, and continue to cook five minutes more for medium doneness.

Slice the steak against the grain into ¼-inch-thick strips.

Serve with salsa on the side.

• MINI MEATLOAF •

SERVINGS: 4

½ pound ground chuck (90% lean)

½ pound ground turkey

1 egg, lightly beaten, or ¼ cup Egg Beaters

2 tablespoons tomato paste

¼ cup minced onion

¼ cup minced carrot

¼ cup minced celery

1 tablespoon of your favorite dried herbs (thyme, rosemary, parsley, basil, etc.), or a combination

2 tablespoons fresh or dried bread crumbs

Salt and freshly ground black pepper to taste

Preheat the oven to 350°F.

Combine all ingredients in a bowl, mixing with your hands or a wooden spoon until well combined.

Form the mixture into four small loaves.

Bake on a rimmed baking sheet for 35 minutes, or until the juices bubbling around the loaves runs clear.

• BAKED DIJON CHICKEN •

SERVINGS: 2

Two 4-ounce boneless, skinless
   chicken breasts
1 tablespoon light mayonnaise
1 tablespoon country Dijon
   mustard
1 pinch freshly ground black
   pepper

1 pinch ground paprika
2 teaspoons chopped fresh
   parsley
Salt to taste

Trim all visible fat from the chicken.

Pound chicken, between two pieces of waxed paper, with a mallet, until ½ inch thick.

In a small bowl, combine the mayonnaise, mustard, pepper, and paprika.

Place the chicken in a microwave-safe baking dish. Coat one side of the chicken with the mayonnaise mixture and microwave on high for 3 minutes.

Turn the chicken over and coat the other side. Cook for an additional 3 minutes, or until chicken is cooked through and no longer pink.

Sprinkle with the chopped parsley and salt to taste.

· BBQ CHICKEN BREASTS ·

SERVINGS: 2

Two 4-ounce boneless, skinless
  chicken breasts

4 ounces barbecue sauce

Preheat a broiler or grill.

Trim the chicken breast of all visible fat.

In a shallow dish, cover the chicken with the barbecue sauce.

Broil or grill the chicken for 15 to 20 minutes, turning once or twice,
  or until cooked through and no longer pink.

· BAKED HERBED CHICKEN À L'ORANGE ·

SERVINGS: 2

Two 4-ounce boneless, skinless
  chicken breasts
½ cup chicken broth
3 tablespoons white wine

½ teaspoon ground thyme
½ teaspoon dried rosemary
1 medium navel orange, sliced
  thick

Preheat the oven to 375°F.

Trim all visible fat from the chicken breasts.

In a small bowl, whisk the chicken broth, wine, and herbs together.

Place the chicken in a shallow baking dish and pour the wine mixture over them. Place the orange slices on top of the chicken.

Bake for 25 minutes, or until the meat is cooked through and no
  longer pink.

CRUNCHY CHICKEN

SERVINGS: 2

Two 4-ounce boneless, skinless
   chicken breasts
¼ cup 1% milk or buttermilk
⅓ cup Kellogg's Corn Flakes
   cereal

1 pinch garlic powder
1 pinch ground paprika
1 pinch salt
1 pinch ground thyme

Preheat the oven to 375°F.

Trim all visible fat from the chicken breasts.

Dip the chicken in the milk.

Combine the corn flakes and spices in a plastic bag and shake the
   bag to combine.

Add the chicken to the corn flake mixture, shake to coat, remove,
   and place in a baking dish.

Bake for 25 minutes, or until meat is cooked through and no longer
   pink.

• GINGER CITRUS CHICKEN •

SERVINGS: 1

One 4-ounce boneless, skinless
  chicken breast
1 tablespoon orange marmalade
1 teaspoon honey

½ teaspoon country Dijon
  mustard
¼ teaspoon ground ginger
1 pinch chile powder

Preheat a broiler or grill.

Trim all visible fat from the chicken.

Combine the marmalade, honey, mustard, ginger, and chile powder
  in a small bowl. Mix well.

Brush half of the marmalade mixture over the chicken breast.

Broil or grill the chicken for 10 minutes per side, or until juices run
  clear. Brush with the remaining marmalade mixture just before
  serving.

· KICKIN' CHICKEN AND RICE CASSEROLE ·

SERVINGS: 4

1 teaspoon unsalted butter
3 cups cooked brown rice
¾ cup 1% milk
2 eggs, lightly beaten
2 cups shredded cheddar cheese
    (or other cheese, full-fat or low-
    fat)
Two 4-ounce skinless, boneless
    chicken breasts, lightly cooked
    and chopped

⅓ cup finely chopped cilantro
½ cup chopped onion
Salt and/or freshly ground black
    pepper to taste

Preheat the oven to 375°F.

Lightly butter a casserole dish.

Combine the rice, milk, eggs, cheese, chicken, cilantro, and onion
    in the casserole dish and stir thoroughly.

Bake for 45 to 55 minutes.

Season with salt and/or pepper to taste.

· BEAN, RICE, AND CHICKEN STEW ·

SERVINGS: 2

4 ounces roasted boneless, skinless chicken breast

2 cups cooked brown rice

½ cup cooked black or red beans (canned, rinsed, and drained is fine)

⅛ cup chopped white onion

2 teaspoons ketchup

1 teaspoon Dijon mustard

1 teaspoon Worcestershire sauce

½ teaspoon brown sugar

Preheat the oven to 375°F.

Combine all the ingredients in an oven-safe casserole dish. Mix until all the ingredients are well blended.

Bake, uncovered, for 55 to 60 minutes.

· SPANISH RICE WITH CHICKEN ·

SERVINGS: 4

1 cup white or brown rice

2 cups chicken broth

Two 5-ounce boneless, skinless
chicken breasts

3 teaspoons olive oil

3 cloves garlic, minced

1 small red bell pepper, seeded
and diced

1 cup fresh, frozen, or canned
corn kernels

One 8-ounce can tomato sauce

Salt and freshly ground pepper to
taste

2 teaspoons fresh cilantro

In a large saucepan, bring the rice and chicken broth to a boil. Reduce heat to low, cover, and cook until rice is tender. White rice will take 15 to 20 minutes; brown rice about 45 minutes.

Trim the chicken of all visible fat and sauté it in a skillet with 1 teaspoon oil until cooked through and no longer pink, about 15 minutes.

Remove the chicken and chop it into chunks.

Heat remaining 2 teaspoons oil in the skillet and sauté the garlic, red pepper, and corn for about 5 minutes, stirring occasionally, until pepper is tender.

Add the chicken, pepper and corn mixture, and tomato sauce to the rice, mix, and let simmer, covered, for 10 minutes over low heat.

Add salt and pepper and serve, garnished with the cilantro.

• CHICKEN POT PIE FOLD-OVERS •

SERVINGS: 4

1 small frozen deep-dish pie crust,
    defrosted
3 carrots, peeled and sliced ¼
    inch thick
1 pound boneless, skinless
    chicken breast, cut into 1-inch
    cubes
½ medium onion, sliced

1 teaspoon olive oil
½ cup frozen peas
½ cup low-fat chicken broth
2 tablespoons minced fresh
    tarragon
½ teaspoon flour
Salt and freshly ground pepper to
    taste

Preheat the oven per instructions on the pie crust box.

Boil the carrots in salted water to cover until tender.

Trim all excess fat from chicken. While the carrots cook, sauté the chicken and onion in olive oil over medium-high heat.

Add the carrots, peas, broth, tarragon, flour, and salt and pepper to the sauté pan and cook on medium-low heat until broth is slightly reduced.

Remove the pie crust from its pan, flatten it onto a cookie sheet, and cut it into quarters. Spoon mixture from the sauté pan onto the pie-crust quarters.

Fold over quarters lengthwise, like you're making a paper airplane, and pinch edges.

Pierce top of each fold-over with a fork.

Bake for the length of time indicated on the pie-crust container, or until the crust is brown and the chicken mixture is beginning to bubble through.

· TURKEY FAJITAS ·

SERVINGS: 2

Two 4-ounce turkey breast cutlets
½ tablespoon olive oil
4 slices onion
1 medium green bell pepper,
    seeded and sliced thinly
2 tablespoons light sour cream

2 ounces cheddar cheese,
    shredded (full-fat or low-fat)
2 whole wheat tortillas

Trim the turkey breast of all visible fat.

Slice the turkey into thin strips.

Cook the turkey strips with the oil in a nonstick skillet for 8 minutes, or until lightly browned.

Remove the turkey and set aside. Sauté the onions and pepper in the same skillet until tender. Add the turkey back to the skillet and cook until the turkey is heated through.

To serve, place half of the meat mixture on each tortilla, then top with 1 tablespoon of the sour cream and 1 ounce of the shredded cheese. Roll up the tortillas and serve.

· BLACK AND WHITE CHILI ·

SERVINGS: 4

1 tablespoon extra virgin olive oil
1 pound ground turkey
2 medium onions, chopped
3 cloves garlic, minced
One 15-ounce can cannellini
  beans, rinsed and drained
One 15-ounce can black beans,
  rinsed and drained

One 15-ounce can diced
  tomatoes
2 bay leaves
32 ounces low-fat chicken broth
¼ cup chopped fresh cilantro
1 pinch freshly ground white
  pepper

Heat the olive oil in a large soup pot over medium heat.

Add the turkey, onion, and garlic, and cook until the turkey is
  browned.

Add the beans, tomatoes, bay leaves, and broth, and bring to a boil.
  Reduce heat, and let simmer for 20 minutes.

Add the cilantro and pepper, let simmer for two more minutes, and
  then serve.

· TURKEY CHILI ·

2 pounds ground turkey
½ large onion, chopped
1 teaspoon olive oil
½ bottle (12 ounce) beer (lite or
regular)
Three 15-ounce cans dark red
kidney beans (two cans
unrinsed, one rinsed)

Three 15-ounce cans diced
tomatoes (with liquid)
2 tablespoons chile powder (or to
taste)

Cook turkey and onion in olive oil over medium heat until browned. Mix in beer, beans, tomatoes, and chile powder and cook over medium-low heat for 20 minutes, or until mixture is thickened.

• BAKED FLOUNDER •

SERVINGS: 2

2 tablespoons flour

1 pinch salt

1 pinch freshly ground black
  pepper

Two 4-ounce flounder fillets

Freshly squeezed juice of ½
  lemon

Preheat the oven to 375°F.

Combine the flour, salt, and pepper in a small mixing bowl.

Place fillets in a shallow baking dish. Cover the fillets with the flour
  mixture and the lemon juice.

Bake in the oven for 15 minutes, or until the fish flakes when
  pierced with a fork.

SERVINGS: 2

Two 5-ounce halibut fillets
1 tablespoon lemon juice
1 pinch ground dillweed
1 pinch ground paprika

1 pinch freshly ground black
  pepper
2 large slices tomato (optional)

Place the fillets in a glass or microwave-safe baking dish.

Pour the lemon juice over the fish and sprinkle the seasonings on
the fish.

Cover with plastic wrap and poke holes in the top to vent.

Microwave on high for 2 to 4 minutes, or until the fish flakes when
poked with a fork.

Optional: Top each fillet with a tomato slice before serving.

· GRILLED HALIBUT ·

Two 5-ounce halibut fillets
1 tablespoon olive oil
⅓ cup lemon juice
2 teaspoons country Dijon
    mustard
½ teaspoon ground cumin

1 pinch freshly ground black
    pepper
2 cloves garlic, minced
1 tablespoon chopped fresh
    parsley

Place the halibut in a shallow dish. Combine the olive oil, lemon
    juice, mustard, cumin, pepper, and garlic, and pour over the fish.
Cover and let marinate in the refrigerator for 45 minutes.
Lightly oil and preheat a grill or skillet.
Remove the fish from the marinade and place it on the grill or in the
    skillet. Cook 5 minutes, brush with marinade, and turn.
Cook 5 more minutes. Fish should flake when tested with a fork.
Sprinkle with parsley before serving.

SERVINGS: 2

3 tablespoons cornmeal

1 pinch ground celery seeds

1 tablespoon chopped fresh
   parsley

1 pinch salt

1 pinch freshly ground black
   pepper

Two 5-ounce farmed rainbow trout
   fillets

1 teaspoon olive oil

Mix together the cornmeal, celery seeds, chopped parsley, salt, and
   pepper.

Cover the fish with the cornmeal mixture, pressing it onto both sides
   of the fish.

Heat the olive oil in a nonstick skillet. Cook the fish for 2 to 3 minutes per side. Fish should be brown and crisp and flake when
   pierced with a fork.

• CAJUN RED SNAPPER •

SERVINGS: 2

Two 4-ounce red snapper fillets
½ teaspoon ground cayenne
  pepper

1 teaspoon salted butter, melted
1 tablespoon lemon juice

Heat a heavy skillet (preferably cast iron) over medium-high heat until very hot.

Sprinkle cayenne pepper over both sides of the fish to coat it well.

Cook the fish in the hot pan for 2 to 3 minutes, until the bottom is dark brown.

Drizzle ¼ teaspoon melted butter over each fillet. Turn fish over. Drizzle blackened side of fish with remaining butter. Cook 2 to 3 minutes, until the other side is dark brown.

Drizzle with lemon juice. Serve hot.

· GRILLED SALMON WITH MARINADE ·

SERVINGS: 2

FOR THE MARINADE
⅓ cup white wine
1 clove garlic, minced
1 tablespoon soy sauce
½ teaspoon ground paprika

⅓ cup olive oil
Two 5-ounce salmon fillets
Salt and freshly ground black
    pepper to taste
Half a lemon

To make the marinade: Combine the wine, garlic, soy sauce, paprika, and olive oil, and whisk together.

Marinate the salmon for at least 1 hour before grilling.

Lightly oil and preheat a grill or skillet.

Place the fish on the hot grill or in the skillet and cook for 5 minutes, then turn.

Lower the heat and continue cooking for 5 to 10 minutes, or until fish flakes when tested with a fork.

Sprinkle the fish with salt and pepper and squeeze the lemon juice over it before serving.

· GLAZED HONEY SALMON ·

FOR THE MARINADE

4 tablespoons soy sauce

2 tablespoons whiskey (optional)

2 tablespoons honey

1 tablespoon sesame oil

1 clove garlic, minced

1 teaspoon fresh ginger root,
  grated

Freshly ground black pepper to
  taste

Four 5-ounce salmon fillets, with
  skin

Olive oil or butter spray for grill

Mix the marinade ingredients and marinate the salmon fillets for 30
  minutes in the refrigerator, turning the fish in the marinade once
  or twice.

Spray a grill with olive oil or butter spray and preheat it.

Cook the salmon skin-side down first. After 4 to 6 minutes, remove
  the fish from the skin, turn, and baste with the marinade. Cook
  the second side for 4 to 6 minutes, until it is opaque throughout,
  but don't overcook it.

• BAKED SEA BASS WITH VEGETABLES •

SERVINGS: 2

Two 5-ounce sea bass
   fillets
Salt and freshly ground black
   pepper to taste
1 lemon, halved
1 bunch fresh fennel fronds
1 tablespoon unsalted butter,
   melted
1 small onion, thinly sliced

2 small potatoes, such as
   creamers or Red Bliss, thinly
   sliced
2 tomatoes, quartered
3 tablespoons Pernod liquor
1 tablespoon chopped fresh
   parsley
1 bunch fresh broccoli

Preheat the oven to 375°F.

Season the fish with salt and pepper to taste and the juice of half a lemon. Place the fish in a baking pan.

Cover the fish with the fennel fronds and drizzle with the melted butter.

Place onion and potato slices around the fish and bake at 375°F for 15 minutes.

Add tomatoes, drizzle with Pernod, and bake 5 to 10 minutes more, or until fish flakes easily with a fork.

Sprinkle with parsley and garnish with the remaining lemon half.

Serve with steamed broccoli.

To make the broccoli: Wash the broccoli, separate the florets, and peel and cut up the stems. Place in a steamer basket within a saucepan. Add about 1 inch of water to the bottom of the saucepan. Cover and place on high heat. Bring to a boil and steam for about 8 minutes, or until the broccoli turns bright green and is tender.

· BAKED CRABMEAT EXTRAVAGANZA ·

SERVINGS: 4

Vegetable oil or butter spray for
　greasing dish
1 tablespoon unsalted butter
⅓ cup finely chopped onion
1 pound crabmeat, picked over
　and cartilage removed

1 teaspoon Worcestershire sauce
2 tablespoons country Dijon
　mustard
4 egg whites, beaten with a whisk
　or fork
2 tablespoons Parmesan cheese

Preheat the oven to 375°F. Spray a casserole dish or baking pan
　lightly with vegetable oil or butter spray.

Melt the butter in a saucepan and add the onion. Sauté until onion
　is soft.

Combine the onion, crabmeat, Worcestershire sauce, and mustard.

Add the beaten egg whites. Pour the mixture into the casserole dish
　and sprinkle with the cheese.

Bake for 25 to 30 minutes, or until lightly browned. Remove from
　oven, cut, and serve hot.

· SHRIMP CREOLE BONANZA ·

½ tablespoon olive oil

½ cup chopped celery

¾ cup chopped onion

2 garlic cloves, minced

1 small green bell pepper, chopped

1 small red bell pepper, chopped

1 teaspoon Worcestershire sauce

1 tablespoon lemon juice

1 8-ounce can tomato sauce

1 pound fresh or frozen shrimp, peeled and deveined

1 pinch salt

1 pinch freshly ground black pepper

1 cup cooked brown rice

Heat the oil in a saucepan and add the celery, onion, garlic, peppers, Worcestershire sauce, and lemon juice.

Sauté, stirring occasionally, until vegetables are tender, about 8 to 10 minutes.

Pour in the tomato sauce and shrimp. Cover and cook for 10 to 15 minutes over medium heat. Season with the salt and pepper.

Serve the shrimp over brown rice.

• ROASTED BUTTERNUT SQUASH • WITH CREAMY CHEESE SAUCE

SERVINGS: 4

1 large butternut squash
½ teaspoon salt
2 tablespoons olive oil
1 teaspoon ground dried sage
⅛ teaspoon freshly ground black
   pepper

FOR THE SAUCE
½ cup 1% milk
1 cup grated cheddar cheese (full-
   fat or low-fat)
½ teaspoon salt

3 scallions, chopped

Preheat the oven to 425°F.

Peel the squash, cut in half lengthwise, seed, and dice into ½-inch
   pieces.

Toss the squash with the salt, oil, sage, and pepper.

Spread the squash on a baking sheet.

Roast for 30 minutes, stirring periodically.

Make the sauce: While the squash is roasting, heat the milk until almost at a boil. Mix in the cheddar cheese and salt and stir until
   cheese is melted. Keep warm.

When the squash is tender and starts to turn brown, turn the squash
   into a bowl and top with the sauce and the scallions.

• SUGAR-GLAZED CARROTS WITH HERBS •

SERVINGS: 4

2 cups carrots, peeled and sliced
    into rounds
1 teaspoon chopped fresh basil
2 tablespoons chopped fresh
    parsley

1 tablespoon unsalted butter
2 tablespoons sugar

Preheat the oven to 400°F.

Boil the carrots until soft in boiling salted water (about 5 minutes).

Combine the basil and parsley and spread half of it on a buttered baking pan. Add the carrots, then top with the remainder of herbs and the sugar.

Bake for 10 minutes, or until carrots are tender.

SERVINGS: 4

2 tablespoons olive oil

2 cups fresh or frozen cauliflower florets

1 cup fresh or frozen sliced carrots

One 10-ounce package frozen peas

½ teaspoon salt

¼ teaspoon freshly ground black pepper

1 tablespoon chopped pimiento

Heat the oil in a skillet over low heat. Add the cauliflower and carrots and sauté for 10 minutes, stirring occasionally.

Add peas, salt, and pepper. Cook 10 minutes longer.

Add the pimiento and serve.

SERVINGS: 4

1 bunch (1 pound) collard greens

⅓ medium head cabbage,
  coarsely shredded

2 tablespoons olive oil

1 clove garlic, minced

1 medium white onion, sliced

2 teaspoons rice vinegar

Rinse the collards, remove and discard stems, and slice into ribbons.

Bring 3 quarts water to a boil in a large pot. Add the collard greens, return to a boil, and cook 4 minutes, or until the greens are tender-crisp. Remove the greens with a slotted spoon to a colander, leaving the water in the pot.

Return the water to a boil, add the cabbage, and cook for 1 minute. Pour into the colander and let drain.

In a large skillet, heat the olive oil over medium-low heat. Sauté the garlic and onion for 5 minutes, or until softened. Add the greens and cabbage and sauté 3 minutes, stirring. Add the vinegar.

Toss and serve immediately.

· STUFFED GRILLED PEPPERS ·

3 tablespoons olive oil
¼ teaspoon dried oregano
2 tablespoons chopped fresh
 basil
1 pinch red pepper flakes
3 cloves garlic, minced
1 small zucchini, chopped
2 cups cooked brown rice
Salt and freshly ground black
 pepper to taste

2 large red bell peppers, halved
 lengthwise, cores and seeds
 removed
¾ cup mozzarella cheese (full-fat
 or low-fat), shredded
1 pinch ground paprika

Preheat the oven to 375°F.

Heat 1 tablespoon of the olive oil, oregano, basil, red pepper flakes, garlic, and zucchini in a saucepan and sauté for 5 minutes, stirring occasionally. Do not let the garlic burn.

Add the rice and sauté a few more minutes, until heated through.

Season with the salt and pepper.

Rub the pepper halves with 1 tablespoon olive oil.

Scoop the rice mixture into the pepper halves. Sprinkle the mozzarella cheese on top, and drizzle with the remaining olive oil.

Bake uncovered, until peppers are tender, approximately 45 minutes.

Sprinkle with paprika and serve hot.

SERVINGS: 4

Cooking spray for a grill
2 red bell peppers, seeded and
    quartered
2 yellow bell peppers, seeded and
    quartered
12 asparagus spears
1 small eggplant, cut in quarters
    lengthwise
1 medium zucchini, cut in quarters
    lengthwise

1 yellow squash, cut in quarters
    lengthwise
6 plum tomatoes
2 tablespoons extra virgin olive oil
½ teaspoon freshly ground black
    pepper
¼ teaspoon salt
⅓ cup fat-free or low-fat Italian or
    ranch dressing

Spray a grill with cooking spray and preheat it.

Brush the vegetables with the olive oil and sprinkle them evenly
    with black pepper and salt. Place the bell peppers on the grill;
    cook for 5 minutes, turning as needed. Continue to cook, turning,
    as you add the remaining vegetables in the following order.

Add the eggplant and grill 3 minutes, turning.

Add the asparagus and grill 3 minutes, turning.

Add the zucchini and yellow squash and grill 3 minutes, turning.

Add the tomatoes and grill 3 minutes, turning, or until all vegetables
    are tender.

Drizzle with the dressing before serving.

· GINGER SNAPPING STEAMED VEGETABLES ·

2 medium carrots, peeled and
   sliced into ¼-inch-thick
   rounds
1 cup cauliflower florets, fresh or
   frozen

1 cup broccoli florets, fresh or
   frozen
2 small zucchini, sliced into
   ½-inch-thick rounds
1-inch piece fresh ginger root,
   julienned

In the bottom of a saucepan, place a steamer basket and water to a
   depth of 1 inch. Bring to a boil. Layer the steamer basket, in order, with carrots, cauliflower, broccoli, zucchini, and ginger root.
   Cover and steam 5 to 7 minutes, or until barely tender.
Remove the steamer basket from the saucepan. Remove the ginger
   root.
Pour vegetables into a serving dish and serve immediately.

· RED BEANS AND RICE ·

1 tablespoon olive oil
1 small green bell pepper,
    chopped
1 large onion, chopped
½ cup minced celery
Two 15-ounce cans dark red
    kidney beans (undrained)
1 teaspoon chile powder
2 teaspoons Worcestershire
    sauce

2 ounces pimiento, chopped
One 11-ounce can tomato paste
3 tablespoons ketchup
2 cups cooked brown rice
2 tablespoons chopped fresh
    parsley
½ cup chopped scallion

Heat a saucepan over medium-high heat, add oil, and sauté pepper, onion, and celery until soft, approximately three minutes.

Add the beans and remaining ingredients, except the brown rice, parsley, and scallions.

Bring to a boil. Cover and simmer over low heat for 35 minutes.

Serve the bean mixture over the rice, garnished with the parsley and scallion.

· CREAMY SUCCOTASH ·

SERVINGS: 4

One 15-ounce can lima beans,
    drained
½ teaspoon salt
1 pinch freshly ground black
    pepper

One 15-ounce can corn (not
    creamed)
3 teaspoons flour
½ cup 1% milk

Cook the lima beans in ½ cup water seasoned with the salt and pepper for 8 to 10 minutes.

Add the corn and bring mixture to a boil. Reduce the heat, cover, and cook 5 additional minutes.

Whisk the flour into the milk, and gradually stir the mixture into the vegetables. Cook, stirring, until thickened.

· GRANDMA'S VEGETABLE STEW ·

SERVINGS: 4

2 tablespoons unsalted butter

2 tablespoons extra virgin olive oil

1 large onion, chopped

1 clove garlic, minced

8 ounces mushrooms

One 15-ounce can peas

One 16-ounce can whole peeled
  tomatoes

½ medium green pepper,
  chopped

1 cup carrots, chopped

1 cup celery, chopped

1 teaspoon dried oregano

1 teaspoon dried thyme

1 teaspoon dried basil

¼ teaspoon salt

¼ teaspoon freshly ground black
  pepper

Place all ingredients in a large, uncovered pot with 2 cups of hot water and bring to a boil. Reduce heat and cook on low heat for 35 to 45 minutes. Occasionally taste for richness of flavor and correct seasonings.

· WILD RICE PILAF ·

SERVINGS: 2

1 cup wild rice

3 cups chicken broth

1½ cups sliced mushrooms

1½ cups diced celery

One 10-ounce package artichoke
hearts, frozen

¼ cup sliced scallion

2 tablespoons extra virgin olive oil

1 teaspoon grated lemon peel

1 tablespoon lemon juice

½ teaspoon dried thyme

Freshly ground black pepper to
taste

Preheat the oven to 375°F.

Combine the rice with 2½ cups of chicken broth in a saucepan, and
bring to a boil. Reduce to simmer, cover, and cook for 30 minutes.
Don't drain.

Sauté the mushrooms, celery, artichoke hearts, and scallion in the
olive oil, stirring occasionally, until the vegetables are tender,
about 10 to 15 minutes. Mix in the remaining ingredients, combine with the rice mixture, and place in a shallow 2-quart casserole dish.

Bake for 30 to 40 minutes.

• TOMATO SALSA •

MAKES 3 CUPS

5 tomatoes, diced

4 cloves garlic, minced

2 teaspoons salt

2 ounces fresh basil leaves, snipped with scissors into thin ribbons, or 2 ounces cilantro leaves, minced

1 jalapeño pepper, seeded and minced (or more if you like it hot)

¼ cup extra virgin olive oil

1 teaspoon freshly ground black pepper

Place the tomatoes in a mixing bowl and combine with the garlic, salt, basil or cilantro, jalapeño, oil, and pepper.

Let marinate at room temperature for 20 minutes.

· MANGO SALSA ·

1 large mango, peeled, pitted, and
diced
1/3 cup diced red onion
1/4 cup diced red bell pepper
1 jalapeño pepper, seeded and
minced

1 teaspoon red wine vinegar
1/2 teaspoon sugar
2 tablespoons fresh mint or
cilantro, chopped
1 tablespoon lime juice

Combine all ingredients in a bowl and chill for at least 30 minutes.
Serve over chicken, fish, or grilled vegetables.

• APPLE AND BANANA SMOOTHIE •

SERVINGS: 1

½ cup orange juice (not from
   concentrate)
6 cubes ice
¼ cup 1% milk or soy milk

1 banana, peeled and sliced
1 red apple, peeled, cored, and
   chopped into small chunks
3 teaspoons plain low-fat yogurt

Place all ingredients in a blender and process until smooth, approximately 20 seconds. Serve in a glass.

• BERRY FRUITY SMOOTHIE •

SERVINGS: 2

½ cup raspberries
½ cup blackberries
⅓ cup nonfat vanilla yogurt
1 cup orange juice (not from
  concentrate)

6 cubes ice
1 small banana, peeled and
  sliced

Place all ingredients in a blender and process until smooth. Serve in
  a glass.

· EXOTIC FRUIT SMOOTHIE ·

SERVINGS: 2

1 papaya, peeled, seeded, and
chopped

1 mango, peeled, pitted, and
chopped

½ cup blueberries

½ cup strawberries

3 ounces low-fat yogurt

6 ice cubes

Place all ingredients in a blender and process until smooth. Serve in a glass.

· ORANGE FUSION SMOOTHIE ·

SERVINGS: 2

1 small banana, peeled and sliced

1 peach, peeled, halved, pitted, and cut into cubes

1 cup raspberries

⅓ cup low-fat yogurt

½ cup orange juice (not from concentrate)

6 ice cubes

Place all ingredients in a blender and process until smooth. Serve in a glass.

• STRAWBERRY-BANANA SMOOTHIE •

SERVINGS: 2

1 banana, peeled and sliced

8 strawberries (without stems)

6 ice cubes

1 scoop nonfat vanilla frozen
yogurt

1 cup 1% or skim milk

1 teaspoon honey

1 tablespoon flaxseed oil
(optional)

Place all ingredients in a blender and process until smooth. Serve in
a glass.

SERVINGS: 2

1 small banana, peeled and sliced
1 large mango, peeled, seeded, and chopped
2 cups orange juice (not from concentrate)

3 ounces fat-free vanilla frozen yogurt
6 ice cubes

Put all ingredients in a blender and process until smooth. Serve in a glass.

APPENDIX

BODY MASS INDEX (BMI)

FIBER CONTENT OF FOODS

HOW TO READ A FOOD LABEL

CALORIC EXPENDITURE DURING VARIOUS ACTIVITIES

BODY MASS INDEX (*BMI*)

	18	19	20	21	22	23	24	25	26	27	28	29	30	31	32	33	34	35	36	37	38	39	40
Height									Body Weight (pounds)														
4'10"	86	91	96	100	105	110	115	119	124	129	134	138	143	148	153	158	162	167	172	177	181	186	191
4'11"	89	94	99	104	109	114	119	124	128	133	138	143	148	153	158	163	168	173	178	183	188	193	198
5'0"	92	97	102	107	112	118	123	128	133	138	143	148	153	158	163	168	174	179	184	189	194	199	204
5'1"	95	100	106	111	116	122	127	132	137	143	148	153	158	164	169	174	180	185	190	195	201	206	211
5'2"	98	104	109	115	120	126	131	136	142	147	153	158	164	169	175	180	186	191	196	202	207	213	218
5'3"	102	107	113	118	124	130	135	141	146	152	158	163	169	175	180	186	191	197	203	208	214	220	225
5'4"	105	110	116	122	128	134	140	145	151	157	163	169	174	180	186	192	197	204	209	215	221	227	232
5'5"	108	114	120	126	132	138	144	150	156	162	168	174	180	186	192	198	204	210	216	222	228	234	240
5'6"	112	118	124	130	136	142	148	155	161	167	173	179	186	192	198	204	210	216	223	229	235	241	247
5'7"	115	121	127	134	140	146	153	159	166	172	178	185	191	198	204	211	217	223	230	236	242	249	255
5'8"	118	125	131	138	144	151	158	165	171	177	184	190	197	203	210	216	223	230	236	243	249	256	262
5'9"	122	128	135	142	149	155	162	169	176	182	189	196	203	209	216	223	230	236	243	250	257	263	270
5'10"	126	132	139	146	153	160	167	174	181	188	195	202	209	216	222	229	236	243	250	257	264	271	278
5'11"	129	136	143	150	157	165	172	179	186	193	200	208	215	222	229	236	243	250	257	265	272	279	286
6'0"	132	140	147	154	162	169	177	184	191	199	206	213	221	228	235	242	250	258	265	272	279	287	294
6'1"	136	144	151	159	166	174	182	189	197	204	212	219	227	235	242	250	257	265	272	280	288	295	302
6'2"	141	148	155	163	171	179	186	194	202	210	218	225	233	241	249	256	264	272	280	287	295	303	311
6'3"	144	152	160	168	176	184	192	200	208	216	224	232	240	248	256	264	272	279	287	295	303	311	319
6'4"	148	156	164	172	180	189	197	205	213	221	230	238	246	254	263	271	279	287	295	304	312	320	328
6'5"	151	160	168	176	185	193	202	210	218	227	235	244	252	261	269	277	286	294	303	311	319	328	336
6'6"	155	164	172	181	190	198	207	216	224	233	241	250	259	267	276	284	293	302	310	319	328	336	345

UNDERWEIGHT	HEALTHY WEIGHT	OVERWEIGHT	OBESE
(<18.5)	(18.5–24.9)	(25–29.9)	(≥30)

Find your height along the left-hand column and look across the row until you find the number that is closest to your weight. The number at the top of that column identifies your BMI.

Source: From A. Must, G. E. Dallal, and W. H. Dietz, "Reference Data for Obesity: 85th and 95th Percentiles of Body Mass Index (wt/ht²) and Triceps Skinfold Thickness." *American Journal of Clinical Nutrition* 53 (1991): 839–846. Adapted with permission by the *American Journal of Clinical Nutrition*, © *American Journal of Clinical Nutrition*, American Society for Clinical Nutrition.

FIBER CONTENT OF FOODS

To consume more fiber, eat more whole fruits and vegetables, whole grains, and beans. Nuts are also rich in fiber, but they are energy dense, so eat them in small amounts. Use the following list to guide your food choices. It is adapted from research conducted by the Tufts University School of Medicine in Boston and published in the *Tufts Health & Nutrition Letter*.

FRUITS*	GRAMS OF FIBER
Apple (with skin)	4
Banana	3
Blueberries, ½ cup	2
Cantaloupe, 1 cup diced	1
Dates, ⅛ cup dry, chopped	2
Grapefruit, ½	2
Grapes, 1 cup	2
Nectarine (with skin)	2
Orange	3
Peach (with skin)	2
Pear (with skin)	4
Plum (with skin)	1
Prunes (dried), 10	2
Raisins, ⅛ cup	1
Raspberries, ½ cup	4
Strawberries, ½ cup	2
Watermelon, 1 cup diced	1

VEGETABLES†	GRAMS OF FIBER
Broccoli, ½ cup cooked, chopped	2
Broccoli, ½ cup chopped	1

*All values are for 1 medium-size fruit unless otherwise indicated.

†All values are for raw, uncooked vegetables unless otherwise indicated.

Brussels sprouts, ½ cup cooked	3
Carrot, 1 medium	2
Carrots, ½ cup cooked	3
Cauliflower, ½ cup cooked	2
Celery, 1 stalk	1
Corn, ½ cup cooked	2
Cucumber, ½ cup sliced	0.5
French fries, 1 small (2.5 ounces) serving	2
Green beans, ½ cup cooked (frozen)	2
Iceberg lettuce, 1 cup shredded	1
Peas, ½ cup cooked (frozen)	4
Peppers, ½ cup chopped	1
Potato, baked, with skin	5
Potato, baked, without skin	2
Potato, ½ cup mashed	2
Romaine lettuce, 1 cup shredded	1
Spinach, ½ cup chopped	1
Spinach, ½ cup cooked (frozen)	3
Sweet potato, baked with skin	3
Tomato, 1 medium	1

GRAINS, LEGUMES* (BEANS, CHICKPEAS, LENTILS, LIMA BEANS), AND NUTS

	GRAMS OF FIBER
Black beans, ½ cup	8
Bread, 1 slice, white	1
Bread, 1 slice, whole-wheat	2
Bran muffin, 1 medium	3

*Values are for canned or cooked beans.

(Grains, Legumes, and Nuts, continued)	GRAMS OF FIBER
Chickpeas, ½ cup	5
Kidney beans, ½ cup	7
Lentils, ½ cup	8
Lima beans, ½ cup	6
Oatmeal, 1 cup cooked	4
Pasta, ½ cup cooked	1
Peanuts, ½ cup	6
Peanut butter, 2 tablespoons, chunky	2
Popcorn, 3 cups air-popped	2
Rice, 1 cup cooked, white	1
Rice, 1 cup cooked, brown	2
Sesame seeds, 2 tablespoons	1
Sunflower seeds, ⅛ cup	2
Tortilla chips, 1 cup (1.5 oz.)	1
Walnuts, ¼ cup chopped	2
Wheat germ, ¼ cup	4

Source: "Fact Sheet No. 9.333," Table 2, Colorado State University Cooperative Extension.

HOW TO READ A FOOD LABEL

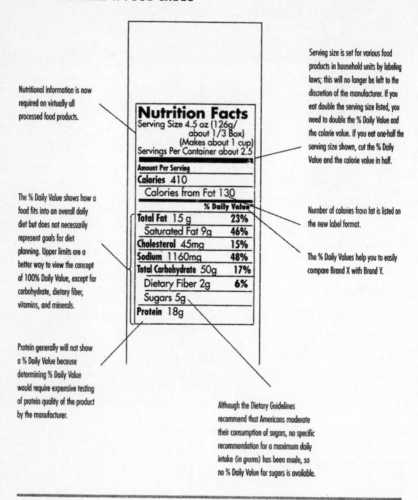

Nutritional information is now required on virtually all processed food products.

The % Daily Value shows how a food fits into an overall daily diet but does not necessarily represent goals for diet planning. Upper limits are a better way to view the concept of 100% Daily Value, except for carbohydrate, dietary fiber, vitamins, and minerals.

Protein generally will not show a % Daily Value because determining % Daily Value would require expensive testing of protein quality of the product by the manufacturer.

Serving size is set for various food products in household units by labeling laws; this will no longer be left to the discretion of the manufacturer. If you eat double the serving size listed, you need to double the % Daily Value and the calorie value. If you eat one-half the serving size shown, cut the % Daily Value and the calorie value in half.

Number of calories from fat is listed on the new label format.

The % Daily Values help you to easily compare Brand X with Brand Y.

Although the Dietary Guidelines recommend that Americans moderate their consumption of sugars, no specific recommendation for a maximum daily intake (in grams) has been made, so no % Daily Value for sugars is available.

Nutrition Facts
Serving Size 4.5 oz (126g/
about 1/3 Box)
(Makes about 1 cup)
Servings Per Container about 2.5

Amount Per Serving

Calories 410

Calories from Fat 130

	% Daily Value*
Total Fat 15 g	23%
Saturated Fat 9g	46%
Cholesterol 45mg	15%
Sodium 1160mg	48%
Total Carbohydrate 50g	17%
Dietary Fiber 2g	6%
Sugars 5g	
Protein 18g	

The Nutrition Facts panel on a current food label. The box is broken into two parts: A is the top, and B is the bottom. The % Daily Value listed on the label is the percentage of the generally accepted amount of a nutrient needed daily that is present in 1 serving of the product. You can use the % Daily Values to compare your diet with current nutrition recommendations for certain diet components. Let's consider dietary fiber. Assume that you consume 2,000 kcal. per day, which is the energy intake corresponding to the % Daily Values listed on labels. If the total % Daily Value for dietary fiber in all the foods you eat in one day adds up to 100%, your diet meets the recommendations for dietary fiber.

Many vitamin and mineral amounts no longer need to be listed on the nutrition label. Only Vitamin A, Vitamin C, calcium, and iron remain. The interest in or risk of deficiencies of the other vitamins and minerals is deemed too low to warrant inclusion.

Some % Daily Value standards, such as grams of total fat, increase as energy intake increases. The % Daily Values on the label are based on a 2,000-kcal. diet. This is important to note if you don't consume at least 2,000 kcal. per day.

Labels on larger packages may list the number of calories per gram of fat, carbohydrate, and protein.

Ingredients, listed in descending order by weight, will appear here or in another place on the package. The sources of some ingredients, such as certain flavorings, will be stated by name to help people better identify ingredients that they avoid for health, religious, or other reasons.

| Vitamin A 10% • Vitamin C 0% |
| Calcium 30% • Iron 15% |

Percent Daily Values are based on a 2,000 calorie diet. Your daily values may be higher or lower depending on your calorie needs:

		Calories: 2,000	2,500
Total Fat	Less than	65g	80g
Sat Fat	Less than	20g	25g
Cholest	Less than	300mg	300mg
Sodium	Less than	2,400mg	2,400mg
Total Carb		300g	375g
Fiber		25g	30g

Calories per gram:
Fat 9 • Carbohydrate 4
• Protein 4

INGREDIENTS: WATER, ENRICHED MACARONI (ENRICHED FLOUR [NIACIN, FERROUS SULFATE (IRON], THIAMINE MONONITRATE AND RIBOFLAVIN], EGG WHITE), FLOUR, CHEDDAR CHEESE (MILK, CHEESE CULTURE, SALT, ENZYME), SPICES, MARGARINE (PARTIALLY HYDROGENATED SOYBEAN OIL, WATER, SOY LECITHIN, MONO- AND DIGLYCERIDES, BETA CARO- TENE FOR COLOR, VITAMIN A PALMITATE), AND MALTODEXTRIN.

Source: Wardlaw, Gordon M., *Contemporary Nutrition*, 4th ed. (New York: McGraw Hill Companies, Inc., 2000).

CALORIC EXPENDITURE
DURING VARIOUS ACTIVITIES

ACTIVITY	CAL/MIN*
Sleeping	1.2
Resting in bed	1.3
Sitting, normally	1.3
Sitting, reading	1.3
Lying, quietly	1.3
Sitting, eating	1.5
Sitting, playing cards	1.5
Standing, normally	1.5
Classwork, lecture (listening)	1.7
Conversing	1.8
Personal toilet	2.0
Sitting, writing	2.6
Standing, light activity	2.6
Washing and dressing	2.6
Washing and shaving	2.6
Driving a car	2.8
Washing clothes	3.1
Walking indoors	3.1
Shining shoes	3.2
Making bed	3.4
Dressing	3.4
Showering	3.4
Driving motorcycle	3.4

*Depends on efficiency and body size. Add 10 percent for each 15 lb. over 150; subtract 10 percent for each 15 lb. under 150.

ACTIVITY	CAL/MIN
Metalworking	3.5
House painting	3.5
Cleaning windows	3.7
Carpentry	3.8
Farming chores	3.8
Sweeping floors	3.9
Plastering walls	4.1
Repairing trucks and automobiles	4.2
Ironing clothes	4.2
Farming, planting, hoeing, raking	4.7
Mixing cement	4.7
Mopping floors	4.9
Repaving roads	5.0
Gardening, weeding	5.6
Stacking lumber	5.8
Sawing with chain saw	6.2
Working with stone, masonry	6.3
Working with pick and shovel	6.7
Farming, haying, plowing with horse	6.7
Shoveling (miners)	6.8
Shoveling snow	7.5
Walking down stairs	7.1
Chopping wood	7.5
Sawing with crosscut saw	7.5–10.5
Tree felling (ax)	8.4–12.7
Gardening, digging	8.6
Walking up stairs	10.0–18.0
Playing pool or billiards	1.8
Canoeing, 2.5 mph–4.0 mph	3.0–7.0

ACTIVITY	CAL/MIN
Playing volleyball, recreational to competitive	3.5–8.0
Golfing, foursome to twosome	3.7–5.0
Pitching horseshoes	3.8
Playing baseball (except pitcher)	4.7
Playing Ping-Pong or table tennis	4.9–7.0
Practicing calisthenics	5.0
Rowing, pleasure to vigorous	5.0–15.0
Cycling, easy to hard	5.0–15.0
Skating, recreational to vigorous	5.0–15.0
Practicing archery	5.2
Playing badminton, recreational to competitive	5.2–10.0
Playing basketball, half or full court (more for fast break)	6.0–9.0
Bowling (while active)	7.0
Playing tennis, recreational to competitive	7.0–11.0
Waterskiing	8.0
Playing soccer	9.0
Snowshoeing (2.5 mph)	9.0
Slide board	9.0–13.0
Playing handball or squash	10.0
Mountain climbing	10.0–15.0
Skipping rope	10.0–15.0
Practicing judo or karate	13.0
Playing football (while active)	13.3
Wrestling	14.4
Skiing	
Moderate to steep	8.0–20.0

ACTIVITY	CAL/MIN
Downhill racing	16.5
Cross-country; 3–10 mph	9.0–20.0
Swimming	
Leisurely	6.0
Crawl, 25–50 yd/min.	6.0–12.5
Butterfly, 50 yd/min.	14.0
Backstroke, 25–50 yd/min.	6.0–12.5
Breaststroke, 25–50 yd/min.	6.0–12.5
Sidestroke, 40 yd/min.	11.0
Dancing	
Modern, moderate to vigorous	4.2–5.7
Ballroom, waltz to rumba	5.7–7.0
Square	7.7
Walking	
Road or field (3.5 mph)	5.6–7.0
Snow, hard to soft (2.5–3.5 mph)	10.0–20.0
Uphill, 15 percent grade (3.5 mph)	8.0–15.0
Downhill, 5–10 percent grade (2.5 mph)	3.5–3.7
15–20 percent grade (2.5 mph)	3.7–4.3
Hiking, 40-lb. pack (3.0 mph)	6.8
Running	
12-min. mile (5 mph)	10.0
8-min. mile (7.5 mph)	15.0
6-min. mile (10 mph)	20.0
5-min. mile (12 mph)	25.0

Source: Sharkey, Brian J., PhD., *Fitness and Health,* 4th ed. (Champaign: Human Kinetics, 1997).

Index

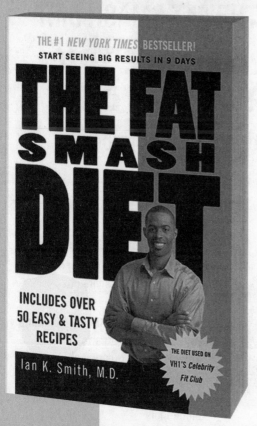

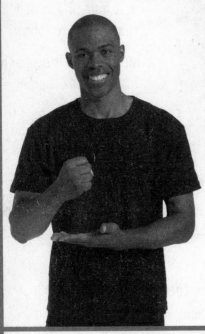